1985
W. B. SAUNDERS COMPANY
Philadelphia ○ London ○ Toronto ○
Mexico City ○ Rio de Janeiro ○
Sydney ○ Tokyo

CW00369284

Pharmacokinetics in Clinical Practice

David J. Greenblatt, M.D.

Professor of Psychiatry and
Associate Professor of Medicine,
Tufts University School of Medicine
Chief, Division of Clinical Pharmacology,
Tufts-New England Medical Center
Boston, Massachusetts

Richard I. Shader, M.D.

Professor and Chairman,
Department of Psychiatry,
Tufts University School of Medicine
Psychiatrist-in-Chief,
Tufts-New England Medical Center,
Boston, Massachusetts

W. B. Saunders Company: West Washington Square
Philadelphia, PA   19105

1 St. Anne's Road
Eastbourne, East Sussex BN21 3UN, England

1 Goldthorne Avenue
Toronto, Ontario M8Z 5T9, Canada

Apartado 26370—Cedro 512
Mexico 4, D.F., Mexico

Rua Coronel Cabrita, 8
Sao Cristovao Caixa Postal 21176
Rio de Janeiro, Brazil

9 Waltham Street
Artarmon, N.S.W. 2064, Australia

Ichibancho, Central Bldg., 22-1 Ichibancho
Chiyoda-Ku, Tokyo 102, Japan

Library of Congress Cataloging in Publication Data

Greenblatt, David J., 1945–

Pharmacokinetics in clinical practice.

1. Pharmacokinetics.   I. Shader, Richard I., 1935–
II. Title. [DNLM: 1. Drugs—metabolism.   2. Kinetics. QV
38 G798p]

RM301.5.G74 1985   615'.7   84–23620

ISBN 0–7216–1148–6

Pharmacokinetics in Clinical Practice   ISBN 0-7216-1148-6

Last digit is the print number: 9   8   7   6   5   4   3   2   1

Contents

Chapter 1
Introduction 1

Chapter 2
Body Compartments and Volumes of Distribution 7

Chapter 3
Exponential Behavior and the Meaning of Half-Life 13

Chapter 4
Mechanisms of Drug Elimination 21

Chapter 5
Intravenous Injection of Drugs 33

Chapter 6
Oral Administration of Drugs 43

Chapter 7
Intramuscular Injection of Drugs 53

Chapter 8
Chronic Dosage: The Extent of Drug Accumulation 61

Chapter 9
Chronic Dosage: The Rate of Drug Accumulation 69

Chapter 10
Pharmacokinetic and Therapeutic Implications of Active
Metabolites 75

Chapter 11
Binding of Drugs to Serum or Plasma Proteins 81

Chapter 12
Nonlinear Pharmacokinetics 89

Chapter 13
The Use of Serum or Plasma Drug Concentrations in
Clinical Practice 95

Chapter 14
Pharmacokinetic Drug Interactions: An Approach to the
Clinical Problem 105

Chapter 15
Pharmacokinetic Drug Interactions: Mechanisms of Drug
Interaction 111

INDEX 123

1

Introduction

Successful drug therapy of human disease depends in part upon the clinician's ability to choose the proper drug. Favorable therapeutic results are possible or likely if the pharmacologic properties of the drug can cause reversal or attenuation of pathologic processes. On the other hand, favorable outcome is much less likely if the drug does not influence, or worsens, the disease process. In many clinical situations, there is no unequivocal choice between correct and incorrect drug. Most older textbooks and educational programs in therapeutics have focused almost entirely upon the concept of "right drug for the right disease," often called the "pharmacologic basis of therapeutics."

In recent years a second important aspect of therapeutics has received increasing attention. This "pharmacokinetic basis of therapeutics" recognizes that clinicians must do more than simply choose the proper drug. They must also select the dose, route of administration, and frequency of administration that will achieve and maintain a proper drug concentration at the molecular recognition site mediat-

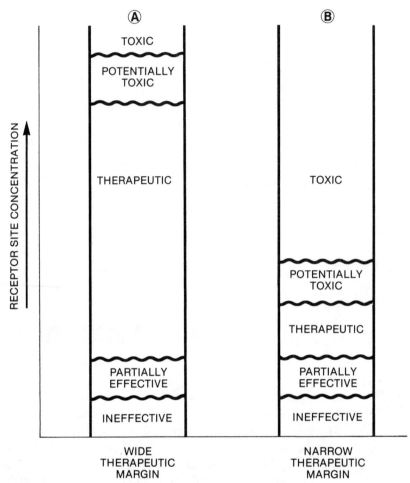

Figure 1–1. Schematic representation of clinical drug effects in relation to concentrations at the receptor site or molecular recognition site mediating clinical action. Drug *A* has a "wide" therapeutic margin (sometimes called a "therapeutic index"), whereas drug *B* has a "narrow" therapeutic margin. For both drugs, progressive increases in receptor site concentrations correspondingly increase clinical effects from ineffective to partially effective, therapeutic, potentially toxic, and finally toxic. For drug *A*, there is a wide range of concentrations which are therapeutic and a correspondingly wide margin between the lower end of the therapeutic range and the beginning of the toxic range. For drug *B*, however, the therapeutic range is narrow, and the margin between therapeutic and toxic concentrations is small. Careful titration of dosage and monitoring of effects therefore is much more important for drug *B* than for drug *A*.

ing clinical action (sometimes called the "receptor site") wherever it exists within the body. If insufficient amounts of drug are present at the site of action, the drug may appear to be ineffective even if it is the "right" drug. Often a drug is discarded for this reason alone, when therapeutic success might have resulted if a proper dose or dosage schedule were chosen. Conversely, the "right" drug may produce toxicity, and be discarded, simply because excessive amounts are present in the body.

The importance of this aspect of therapy for any particular drug depends upon the range, or margin, between its therapeutic and toxic concentrations at the receptor site. This margin is sometimes called the "therapeutic index." For drugs with a wide therapeutic index, a wide range of receptor site concentrations leads to therapeutic success, and potentially toxic concentrations greatly exceed those that are therapeutic (Figure 1–1). Penicillin is one such drug, but other well-documented examples unfortunately are rare. Most drugs have relatively narrow therapeutic margins, and for some (Table 1–1) the difference between toxic and therapeutic amounts is very small indeed. The need for careful titration and monitoring of dosage, clinical effects, and sometimes blood concentrations of drugs listed in Table 1–1 is now widely recognized.

Pharmacokinetics also assumes great importance for those drugs whose time-course and intensity of pharmacologic action parallel those of its concentration in some body fluid. Such drugs include many cardiovascular and anticonvulsant agents, some antibiotics, and certain psychotropic drugs. Understanding how these agents behave in the human body and the relation between clinical effects and drug concentrations in a body fluid (such as blood) can be very valuable when choosing proper dosage schedules and monitoring clinical outcome. On the other hand, understanding the kinetic behavior of certain classes of drugs, such as antineoplastic agents, may not provide complete insight into the time-course of their clinical effects. This is because the net clinical effects of such drugs on the organ or organ

Table 1–1. EXAMPLES OF DRUGS WITH A NARROW THERAPEUTIC MARGIN

Digitalis glycosides
Lithium
Quinidine
Procainamide
Lidocaine
Gentamicin
Phenytoin
Theophylline

systems they are meant to influence seem to bear little relationship to their concentration in any identifiable body fluid.

What is Pharmacokinetics?

"Kinetic" refers to objects in motion. Pharmacokinetics is a discipline that uses mathematical models to describe and predict drug amounts and concentrations in various body fluids and the changes in these quantities over time. For conceptual purposes the behavior of foreign substances within the human body is usually divided, somewhat arbitrarily, into processes of absorption, distribution, biotransformation, and elimination or removal. Each of these processes is assumed to be independent of the others, but in the living organism they necessarily occur simultaneously. The observed time-course of the concentration of a drug in some body fluid is the net result of drug absorption, distribution, biotransformation, and elimination, all of which take place at the same time, at rates that are continuously changing. Not surprisingly, the mathematical framework of pharmacokinetics can become quite complex. Yet the essentials of this discipline can be understood by all persons involved in the use of pharmacologic agents.

The Value of Pharmacokinetics

Understanding and cautious application of pharmacokinetic principles can often assist the clinician in achieving the objective of establishing and maintaining therapeutic yet nontoxic amounts of drugs in the body and at the pharmacologic site of action. More specifically, it can allow a more rational choice of drug doses, frequency of administration, and route of administration. In many cases, identifiable characteristics of the patient and his disease state are known to alter the pharmacokinetic properties of a particular drug within the body (Table 1–2). If appropriate adjustments in drug dosage or frequency of administration can be made to compensate for these kinetic changes, then potential problems of drug ineffectiveness and/or toxicity may be avoided. In a broad sense, the understanding of pharmacokinetics should enhance the likelihood of safe and effective drug therapy.

Table 1–2. FACTORS THAT CAN INFLUENCE THE PHARMACOKINETICS OF DRUGS

Patient Characteristics
Age
Sex
Total body weight
Body habitus
Smoking habits
Alcohol consumption
Other coingested drugs

Disease States
Liver disease (cirrhosis, hepatitis)
Renal disease
Congestive heart failure
Infection
Fever
Shock
Severe burns
Anemia

The Limitations of Pharmacokinetics

Even at its most complex, pharmacokinetics greatly oversimplifies the complicated series of physiologic events that comprise processes such as "absorption" or "elimination." The discipline provides a general framework for understanding drug behavior in the living organism, but it cannot exactly predict how a drug will behave in any particular individual, or how that individual will respond to the drug. Furthermore, for those drugs whose clinical action appears to be unrelated to the time-course of their concentration in any body fluids, pharmacokinetic principles may be of limited value in predicting or understanding clinical effects. Thus, the discipline of pharmacokinetics provides an approach to therapeutics with certain drugs, but it cannot precisely predict individual variations in clinical response and cannot substitute for clinical judgment or careful monitoring and titration of drug effects.

Looking Ahead

This book is designed to provide an outline of pharmacokinetics that can be understood by all those involved in patient care. It is hoped that the limitations as well as the potential value of the discipline will be evident. The ultimate objective is to promote the cause of rational pharmacotherapeutics.

2

Body Compartments and Volumes of Distribution

"Compartments" are a fundamental concept in pharmacokinetics. They represent a simplified but surprisingly useful approach to understanding the processes of drug distribution throughout the living organism. Clinicians should be cautious in interpreting pharmacokinetic compartments since they are *derived from mathematics rather than anatomy or physiology.* Although pharmacokinetic compartments do not correspond to actual anatomic entities, the compartments nonetheless have numeric dimensions of volume (milliliters, liters) as if they were the volume of something real. Understanding drug distribution is made easier if we limit the number of problems that have to be considered simultaneously. For this reason we will assume that all drug doses are given directly into the vascular system by intravenous injection. Drug absorption will be considered in Chapters 6 and 7.

Drug Distribution

Once a drug reaches the vascular system, its passage, or uptake, into any particular body tissue depends upon several factors. The physicochemical properties of the drug are of primary importance. These include the drug's molecular size, the number of polar or charged constitutents it contains, its solubility in aqueous and organic media, and its ability to traverse various types of biomembranes. Drug distribution into a living tissue also depends upon the size of the tissue and the amount of blood flow to it. The concept of compartments and compartmental models has been developed to provide a framework for quantitation of these processes.

Compartments and Volumes

A compartment is an imaginary mathematical space, usually depicted in the pharmacologic literature as a box (Figure 2–1). According to pharmacokinetic theory, when a drug is introduced into a compartment it is rapidly and homogeneously distributed to the entire space. Compartments are often given anatomic designations (such as the "vascular" or the "tissue" compartment), but these correlations are very tenuous and should not be literally accepted. Compartments are also assigned real volumes (in units of liters), but like the compartment themselves, these volumes are fictitious and do not correspond to the actual volume of any one or more body tissues or organs.

Fortunately for the discipline of pharmacokinetics, a "piece" of the body—the blood—is usually available for measurement of drug concentrations. Volumes of compartments are determined by rearranging the definition of concentration, that is

$$\text{Concentration} = \frac{\text{Amount}}{\text{Volume}} \qquad 2.1$$

becomes

$$\text{Volume} = \frac{\text{Amount}}{\text{Concentration}} \qquad 2.2$$

Assume, for example, that the body consists of a single homogeneous compartment (see Figure 2–1). This "one-compartment" model,

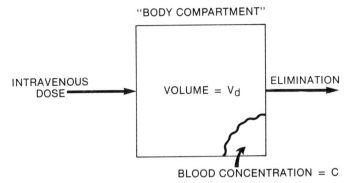

Figure 2–1. Schematic representation of the one-compartment model.

although the simplest of pharmacokinetic models, is surprisingly useful. Further assume that a known dose (D) of a drug is introduced into the body, allowed to distribute throughout the body compartment, and its concentration (C) measured in blood. The volume of the compartment (sometimes called the "apparent volume of distribution" or "Vd") can be determined by substituting the appropriate terms into Equation 2.2 as follows:

$$V_d = \frac{D}{C} \qquad\qquad 2.3$$

Thus, volumes of distribution are simply fictitious proportionality constants that are "cooked up" to explain observed drug concentrations on the basis of the amount of drug known to be present in the body.

Table 2–1 gives examples of apparent volumes of distribution for three benzodiazepine antianxiety agents in the same 70-kilogram human subject, based upon representative data from actual single-dose clinical studies. To make these volumes more generally applicable, they are usually corrected for body weight and expressed in units of liters per kilogram. Note that chlordiazepoxide has the smallest weight-corrected value of V_d, being 0.4 liters per kilogram. Lorazepam has an intermediate value of 1.0 liters per kilogram, and diazepam, at 2.0 liters per kilogram, has the largest. Note that the diazepam appears to distribute itself into a space about twice as large as the body. How can this be? The result reinforces the fictitious nature of compartments and volumes. Clearly, diazepam cannot really be

Table 2–1. VOLUMES OF DISTRIBUTION FOR THREE BENZODIAZEPINE ANTIANXIETY AGENTS AFTER SINGLE INTRAVENOUS DOSES ADMINISTERED TO THE SAME 70-KG SUBJECT

Drug	Intravenous Dose	Blood Concentration after Distribution Is Complete	Apparent Volume of Distribution* (V_d)	Weight-Corrected Volume of Distribution
Chlordiazepoxide	50 mg	1.79 mg/liter	28 liters	0.4 liters/kg
Lorazepam	2 mg	28.6 µg/liter	70 liters	1.0 liters/kg
Diazepam	10 mg	71.4 µg/liter	140 liters	2.0 liters/kg

*Calculated from Equation 2–3.

distributed homogeneously through the body compartment. It must be that diazepam concentrations in some tissues in fact exceed those in blood, giving the appearance of distribution into a space that, if concentrations were uniform throughout, would have to be larger than the body.

Thus, volumes of distribution provide an estimate of the extent of extravascular tissue uptake of drugs. When V_d is small, as for chlordiazepoxide, tissue uptake is limited. Large values of V_d, as with diazepam, indicate extensive tissue distribution. Since many drugs are

Table 2–2. VOLUMES OF DISTRIBUTION FOR REPRESENTATIVE DRUGS IN HUMANS

Drug	Approximate Volume of Distribution (liters per kilogram)
Acetaminophen	1.0
Ampicillin	0.3
Antipyrine	0.6
Cephalexin	0.3
Digoxin	7.0
Furosemide	0.1
Imipramine	15.0
Lidocaine	3.0
Meperidine	3.5
Methotrexate	1.0
Morphine	2.0
Pentobarbital	1.8
Phenytoin	0.6
Procainamide	2.0
Propranolol	3.0
Quinidine	2.3
Theophylline	0.4
Tolbutamide	0.1
Warfarin	0.2

relatively lipid-soluble, extensive tissue uptake and large volumes of distribution tend to be quite common. Table 2–2 gives approximate values of V_d for some commonly used drugs based upon mean values from studies in human subjects. It is important to emphasize that these numbers are only averages. Like other biologic variables, values of V_d for a given drug can vary considerably from person to person and can be influenced by numerous factors such as those described in Table 1–2. Furthermore, knowledge of a drug's pharmacokinetic volume of distribution gives no specific information on the actual sites of distribution. The precise anatomic sites of distribution can be determined only by direct analysis of tissue concentrations, which in turn is usually possible only in animal studies. The very large volume of distribution of digoxin, for example, is explained mainly by extensive uptake into skeletal and cardiac muscle, with relatively little uptake into adipose tissue.

The Two-Compartment Model

Because drug distribution throughout the body does not really occur instantaneously, the one-compartment model does not always adequately explain the observed behavior of drugs. The two-compartment model has been formulated to help understand nonuniform rates of drug distribution (Figure 2–2). The wider applicability of this model unhappily produces greater mathematical complexity.

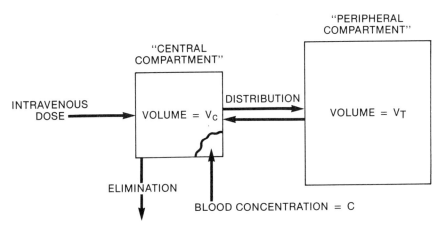

Figure 2–2. Schematic representation of the two-compartment model.

According to this model, the body can be resolved into two compartments, a "central" and a "peripheral" compartment, each of which has its own apparent volume of distribution (often designated as V_c and V_T, respectively). The total apparent volume of distribution of a drug is equal to the sum of V_c and V_T. As suggested before, the compartments often are given anatomic designations, such as the "plasma" and "tissue" compartments, respectively. In many cases it may well be that the central compartment does in fact correspond approximately to the vascular system together with rapidly perfused lean tissues such as heart, liver, lung, kidneys, brain, and endocrine organs, whereas the peripheral compartment corresponds to body fat together with poorly perfused lean tissues (skin, muscle). In general, however, these anatomic and physiologic correlations should be accepted only with caution.

The model further assumes that intravenous doses of drugs are given directly into the central compartment and that all routes of irreversible drug elimination from the body take place via the central compartment (see Chapter 4). Reversible drug distribution takes place between central and peripheral spaces, but the peripheral compartment acts only as a "reservoir." In general, drug distribution tends to occur much more rapidly than drug elimination. Finally, it is usually assumed that a portion of the central compartment (i.e., the blood) is accessible to measurement of concentration of drugs, whereas the peripheral compartment is inaccessible to measurement.

An important consequence of the two-compartment model is that *observed* drug behavior in the body depends upon *both* distribution and elimination. Although the two processes are independent, at no time does one occur without the other. Further implications of the model are discussed in subsequent chapters.

3

Exponential Behavior and the Meaning of Half-Life

If a process of drug absorption, distribution, elimination or biotrans-formation occurred at a constant, fixed rate, then the behavior of a drug over time could be characterized simply by specifying that particular rate. For example, drug elimination would be described in milligrams of the substance eliminated per hour. If 10 milligrams of drug having an elimination rate of 2 milligrams per hour were present in the body at a given point in time, then drug elimination would be complete five hours later. For most drugs, however, changes in their concentrations and amounts in body fluids *do not occur at a single fixed rate*, but rather at rates that change continuously over time. Understanding this type of kinetic behavior is crucial to an overall understanding of pharmacokinetics.

First-Order Processes

The term "first-order" is used to characterize a type of kinetic behavior that fortuitously applies to a large number of drugs. If a process of

13

drug transfer or elimination obeys this first-order model, then the rate of change of drug concentrations over time *varies continuously in relation to the concentration itself.* This concept can be presented in precise mathematical language. Assume that C represents a drug concentration in a body compartment at time t. The quantity $\Delta C/\Delta t$ indicates the rate of change in concentration with time ("Δ" means "change"). These concentration changes per unit time could refer to any of a number of physiologic processes, such as drug removal from the gastrointestinal tract during absorption, drug distribution from blood to tissue, or drug elimination via the kidney or liver. The first-order model assumes that whatever the particular process, $\Delta C/\Delta t$ changes in direct proportion to the drug concentration itself. If k is the proportionality constant between $\Delta C/\Delta t$ and C, then the mathematical formulation of the first-order concept is

$$\frac{\Delta C}{\Delta t} = -kC \qquad\qquad 3.1$$

The quantity k—again, simply a proportionality factor having units of reciprocal time (such as "per hour" or "per second")—is usually called a "rate constant". This is a potentially confusing designation, since k *does not* represent a "constant rate". Note also that a *minus sign* is placed before k in Equation 3.1. This is because drug concentrations in body fluids usually become smaller or decline with time, that is, their rates of change over time are actually negative. The negative sign before the right-hand half of the equation is added to ensure that both sides of the equation have the same sign.

Equation 3.1 indicates that when drug concentrations are high, the *rate* of decline of drug concentrations is also high. At low concentrations, the rate of decline is also low. The rate of drug disappearance varies continuously over time as the concentration itself changes. It is clear why no single rate could possibly characterize such a process.

Exponential Behavior

It is possible to solve Equation 3.1 and determine precisely how drug concentrations vary as a function of time. The solution of Equation

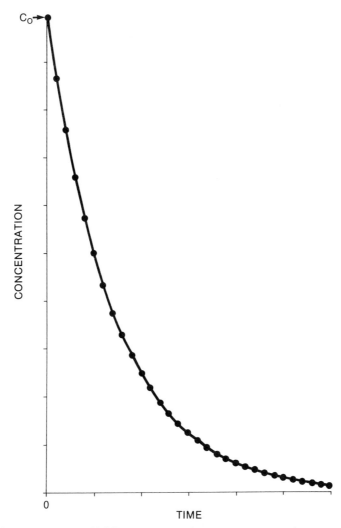

Figure 3–1. "Exponential" fall over time in drug concentrations that are governed by a first-order process. An example is an intravenous bolus dose of a drug into a single body compartment with first-order elimination (see Chapter 2).

3.1 is an *exponential function*. When plotted on a graph, the concentration starts at an initial value (C_o) at time zero, then declines in a curvilinear fashion (Figure 3–1). Clearly, the rate at which the concentration is changing is in itself continuously changing, just as predicted by Equation 3.1. At high drug concentrations, the rate of decline is rapid; at low levels the decline rate is slow. Again, the concentration changes could represent any process that is "first-order," such as the concentration of drug remaining in the gastrointestinal tract after an oral dose, or the drug level in the blood during the elimination process.

First-order, exponential processes, although not describable by a single fixed rate, can be characterized by the concept of half-life (t½). This quantity has units of time and is the *time necessary for the*

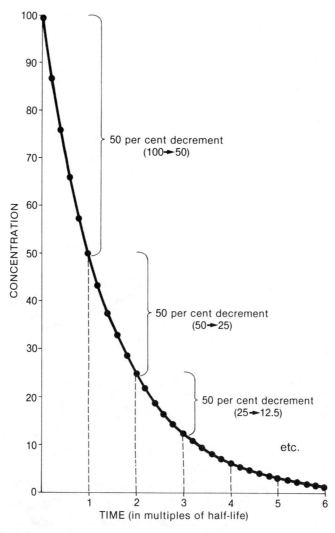

Figure 3–2. The same process as that in Figure 3–1, but with appropriate labels on the time (horizontal) and concentration (vertical) axes. Note that each time a half-life interval elapses, the concentration falls by 50 per cent.

drug concentration to fall by one-half or 50 per cent. Each time an interval equal to a half-life elapses, the concentration falls to one-half of the value at the beginning of that interval.

Assume, for example, that the initial drug concentration (C_o) is 100 units (Figure 3–2). After one half-life has elapsed, the concentration falls by 50 per cent, to 50 units. After another half-life elaspes, the concentration falls by another 50 per cent, this time to 25 units. After the third half-life, it has fallen to 12.5 units, and so on. Notice that the *absolute* amount of change during each half-life interval is *not* the same—it gets smaller as time passes. During the fourth half-life, for example, the absolute change is only 6.25 units—from 12.5 to 6.25—whereas during the first half-life it falls 50 units, from 100 to 50. However, the *percentage* or *ratio* of change is always constant; during *each* half-life that elapses, the concentration falls to 50 per cent or one-half of what it was at the beginning of that interval.

An important fact about *all* first-order processes is that they are *more than 90 per cent complete after four half-life intervals have elapsed.* Note how this applies to Figure 3–2. After four such half-life intervals, the concentration has fallen below 10 units, indicating that whatever process is causing the concentration to decline is more than 90 per cent complete. Note also that in theory *first-order processes are never 100 per cent complete no matter how much time elapses,* any more than the tortoise who successively moves half the remaining distance to the wall will ever reach the wall in a finite number of moves. For practical purposes, however, first-order processes can be considered essentially complete after about eight half-life intervals. Finally, clinicians should be aware that the half-life of a process can be calculated directly from its "rate constant'—designated as *k* in Equation 3.1—as follows:

$$t\frac{1}{2} = \frac{0.693}{k} \hspace{6cm} 3.2*$$

This relationship is of some importance, since pharmacokinetic literature often provides rate constants rather than half-lives of first-order processes.

Figure 3–2 utilizes a vertical or y-axis that is *linear;* that is, equally spaced intervals indicates an arithmetic or linear increase in concen-

---

*The number 0.693 is an approximation of the natural logarithm of 2.

tration (10, 20, 30, 40, 50, . . .). *Semilogarithmic plots* are a different graphic approach commonly used in pharmacokinetics. In such graphs, equally spaced y-axis intervals indicate a geometric (also called exponential or multiplicative) increase in concentration (25, 50, 100, 200, 400, . . .). When plotted on semilogarithmic graphs, first-order processes become straight lines from which it is easy to

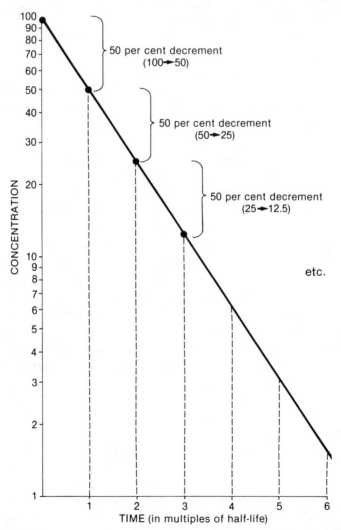

Figure 3–3. The same process as that in Figure 3–2, but plotted with a semilogarithmic concentration axis. This transforms the function into a straight line, from which it is easy to determine half-life. Find any two concentrations that differ by 50 per cent (say, 50 and 25); the time elapsing during this change is the half-life. However, the logarithmic concentration axis distorts the visual image, as described in the text.

determine the half-life (Figure 3–3). On the other hand, the semilog-arithmetic scale causes a misleading visual image: large changes in concentration occurring at the high end of the scale are visually underemphasized because they are "compressed," whereas small changes at the low end are visually "magnified."

Interpreting Half-Life

Characterization of a pharmacokinetic event by a half-life value provides an estimate of how rapidly the process takes place. When a half-life is "short," the event proceeds relatively rapidly. Conversely, a "long" half-life indicates a relatively slow process. In any case, the event is more than 90 per cent completed after four half-life intervals have elapsed. Perhaps the most important pharmacokinetic half-life is that which describes the process of *drug elimination* or removal from the body. This "elimination half-life" (often abbreviated in the literature as $t^{1/2}\beta$) provides insight into how rapidly a drug will disappear from the body after a single dose or after termination of long-term therapy. The elimination half-life also determines the rate at which a drug accumulates and reaches a plateau or "steady-state" level after long-term treatment is initiated. Table 3–1 shows how the elimination half-life of a drug determines how long the drug persists in the body after single doses. It must be emphasized that values of $t^{1/2}$ for a particular drug that are found in reference sources—as well as in Table 3–1—usually are "average" or "representative" values. Like other physiologic and pharmacokinetic events, rates of elimination of any particular drug, and hence values of $t^{1/2}$, will vary from person to person and may be profoundly influenced by such factors

Table 3–1. RELATION OF ELIMINATION HALF-LIFE TO RATES AND AMOUNTS OF DRUG ELIMINATED FROM THE BODY

Multiples of $t^{1/2}$ Elapsed	Per Cent of Dose		Time Elapsed (hr) After Dosage for Drugs Having $t^{1/2}$ Values of:		
	Remaining	Eliminated	3 hours*	15 hours†	48 hours‡
0	100	0	0	0	0
1	50	50	3	15	48
2	25	75	6	30	96
3	12.5	87.5	9	45	144
4	Less than 10	More than 90	12	60	192

*Example: Triazolam.
†Example: Lorazepam.
‡Example: Diazepam.

as those listed in Table 1–2. In fact, t½ for a given drug may vary from time to time even in the same individual.

Drug absorption is another process that often can be characterized by a half-life value (see also Chapter 6). For nearly all drugs, absorption occurs much more rapidly than elimination; hence half-life values for absorption generally are much smaller than those of drug elimination. Drug absorption that appears to be very slow usually results from a chemical characteristic of the molecule itself that causes it to dissolve slowly (as with quinidine gluconate) or from a coating or special matrix construction of the dosage formulation (as with enteric-coated aspirin) to make it a "slow-release" preparation. For most drugs, absorption rates and absorption half-life values tend to be quite variable, both between individuals and from time to time within the same individual. Furthermore, absorption rates can be strongly influenced by such factors as whether the stomach is full or empty, whether other drugs are coadministered, etc.

4

Mechanisms of Drug Elimination

In previous chapters we have discussed "drug elimination" as if drugs were simply removed or extruded from the body or a compartment within the body. This "black box" approach does not describe the actual mechanisms of drug elimination. Living organisms have evolved a system of "defenses" against a variety of foreign chemicals. These systems are both efficient and nonspecific. The vast majority of foreign chemicals that enter a living organism are readily removed in a finite, and usually relatively short, period of time before they may cause harm to some component of the living system. Furthermore, drug elimination mechanisms are surprisingly versatile. They can remove substances to which mammalian systems probably have been exposed throughout evolution (such as certain plant alkaloids) as well as completely new, synthetic chemicals to which no living system has ever been exposed.

Routes of Elimination

Only a small number of routes are available by which *any* substance, whether a foreign chemical or an endogenous product of metabolism, can be ultimately eliminated from the body. Each of these routes has physiologic and physicochemical limitations. The *kidney* obviously provides a means for elimination of water-soluble substances. Most of the kidney's excretory load consists of endogenous compounds (urea, creatinine, etc.) together with small inorganic ions such as sodium, potassium, chloride, and phosphate. Unless a foreign chemical is water-soluble in its unchanged form—and most are not—significant amounts will not be eliminated in the urine. The *feces* are a route of elimination for solid wastes, mainly undigested or unabsorbed components of ingested food. Although cells lining the gastrointestinal tract, particularly the proximal small bowel, are quite efficient in absorbing ingested drugs into the portal blood, the reverse is not true. Drugs seldom re-enter the gastrointestinal tract, whether by mucosal cell secretion or by biliary excretion, in their intact form, and therefore are generally not eliminated intact in the feces unless they were not absorbed to begin with. A third possible route of elimination is the *lungs*. Again, this route has important limitations, since few drugs are volatile enough at body temperature to be exhaled as gases or vapors. Other methods of drug elimination include elimination in sweat, tears, saliva, or breast milk, or permanent fixation to solid tissues such as bone, teeth, or cartilage. Generally these "miscellaneous" routes are not quantitatively important.

It is clear that most foreign chemicals cannot be effectively eliminated intact from the body. The role of the liver is to *transform such chemicals into derivatives that can be more effectively eliminated.*

The Liver

Hepatic biotransformation of drugs generally has the objective of *changing lipid-soluble ("non polar") compounds into water-soluble ("polar") derivatives that can be excreted by the kidney.* A number of transformation mechanisms are available, and most are dependent upon a series of enzymes (termed "microsomal" enzymes) located in cells with the liver. For some drugs more than one molecular transformation is necessary to produce a derivative that can be effectively eliminated. In such cases, some of the metabolic products, or "intermediates," may possess pharmacologic activity. For other drugs only a single biotransformation step is necessary. There are a few exceptions to this general scheme, the most important of which involve ethyl alcohol and chloral hydrate. Hepatic metabolism of these two compounds is dependent upon a different class of enzymes (such as alcohol dehydrogenase) located at a different site within liver cells.

PHASE I REACTIONS

One class of hepatic biotransformation reactions are termed "Phase I" or "preparatory" reactions. These transformations yield intermediate metabolic products that can then undergo the final transformation to highly polar, water-soluble metabolites. Phase I reactions are generally divided into oxidations, reductions, and hydrolyses.

Oxidation. Among the class of oxidation reactions, hydroxylation is one of the most important. Many drugs undergo hydroxylation, rendering themselves susceptible to a subsequent Phase II reaction. Hydroxylation may involve either an aromatic or a nonaromatic substituent (Figure 4–1). Some drugs, such as phenylbutazone, are

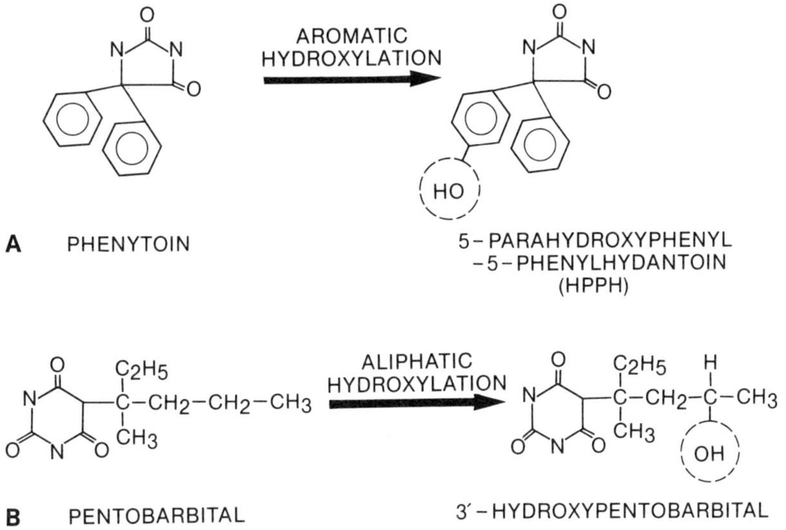

A   PHENYTOIN

AROMATIC HYDROXYLATION

5 – PARAHYDROXYPHENYL –5 – PHENYLHYDANTOIN (HPPH)

B   PENTOBARBITAL

ALIPHATIC HYDROXYLATION

3′ – HYDROXYPENTOBARBITAL

Figure 4–1. Examples of hydroxylation reactions. *A,* Transformation of phenytoin to HPPH by aromatic hydroxylation. *B,* Transformation of pentobarbital to 3′-hydroxypentobarbital by aliphatic hydroxylation.

Table 4–1. PARTIAL LIST OF DRUGS THAT UNDERGO HYDROXYLATION IN HUMANS

| Alprazolam |
| Antipyrine |
| Barbiturates |
| Carbamazepine |
| Desipramine |
| Desmethyldiazepam |
| Digitoxin |
| Glutethimide |
| Ibuprofen |
| Imipramine |
| Midazolam |
| Phenylbutazone |
| Phenytoin |
| Propranolol |
| Quinidine |
| Triazolam |
| Warfarin |

hydroxylated at more than one site on the molecule. Table 4–1 is a partial list of drugs that undergo hydroxylation reactions in humans.

Removal of an alkyl or hydrocarbon group is another common variety of oxidation reaction (Table 4–2). Dealkylation usually involves removal of a substituent attached to a nitrogen or oxygen atom (Figure 4–2) but may also involve an alkyl-substituted sulfur atom. Sulfide oxidation is another oxidative reaction (Figure 4–3), but this is relatively uncommon.

Reduction. Phase I transformations may yield reduction products. Generally such reactions involve nitro substituents, which are then transformed into amino groups (Figure 4–4). In the case of the benzodiazepines nitrazepam and clonazepam, reduction precedes the Phase II acetylation reaction (see p. 26).

Table 4–2. PARTIAL LIST OF DRUGS THAT UNDERGO DEALKYLATION IN HUMANS

| Aminopyrine |
| Amitriptyline |
| Antipyrine |
| Chlordiazepoxide |
| Codeine |
| Diazepam |
| Diphenhydramine |
| Flurazepam |
| Imipramine |
| Lidocaine |
| Meperidine |
| Methamphetamine |
| Phenacetin |
| Prazepam |

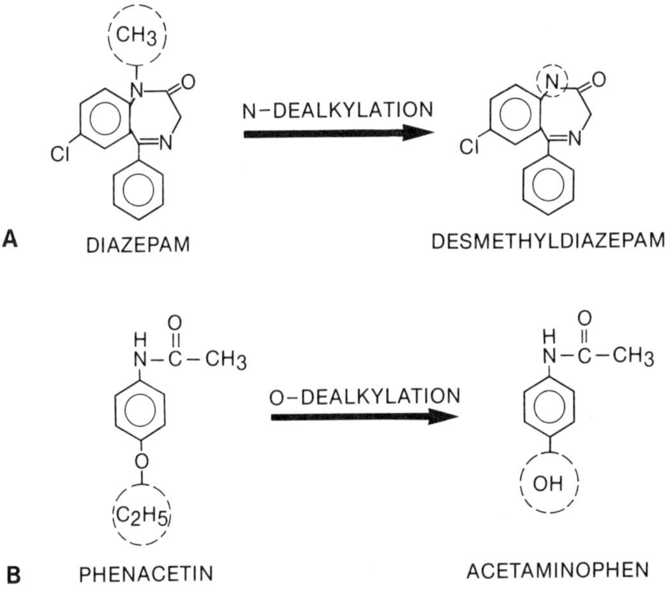

Figure 4–2. Examples of dealkylation reactions. *A,* Transformation of diazepam to desmethyldiazepam by N-dealkylation. *B,* Transformation of phenacetin to acetaminophen by O-dealkylation.

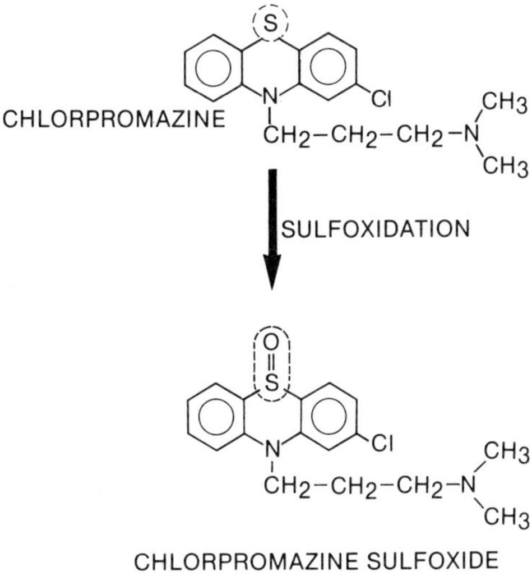

Figure 4–3. Transformation of chlorpromazine to chlorpromazine sulfoxide by sulfoxidation.

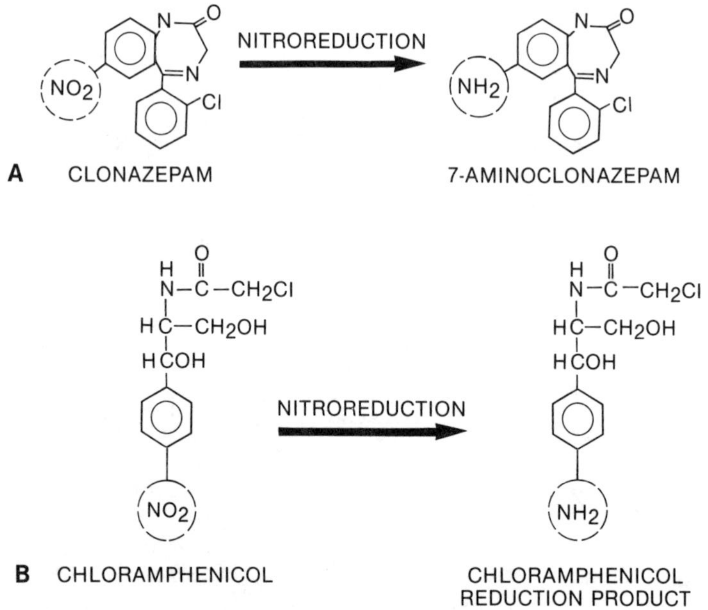

Figure 4–4. Examples of nitroreduction reactions. *A,* Transformation of clonazepam to 7-aminoclonazepam. *B,* Transformation of chloramphenicol to its reduced metabolite.

Hydrolysis. Some molecules are cleaved by a hydrolytic reaction, involving the net addition of a molecule of water. The commonly used analgesic aspirin (acetylsalicylic acid) undergoes hydrolysis as an initial biotransformation step (Figure 4–5).

PHASE II REACTIONS

In some cases, a Phase I reaction renders a drug inactive or allows its excretion. More commonly, a Phase I reaction precedes a final Phase II or "synthetic" biotransformation, yielding a polar, water-soluble metabolite. Conjugation to glucuronic acid is the most common such reaction; some drugs can also be conjugated to sulfuric

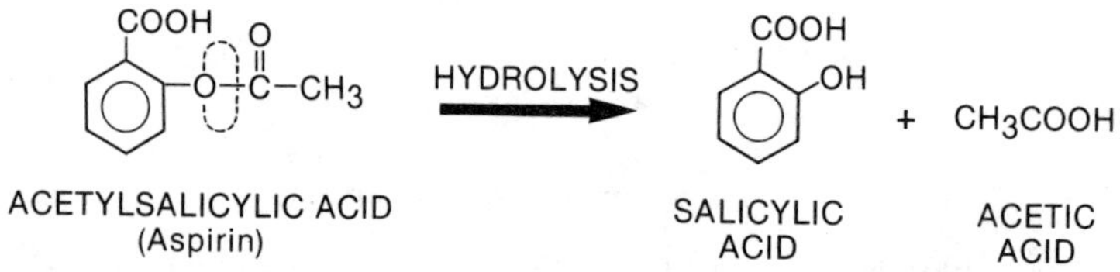

Figure 4–5. Transformation of acetylsalicylic acid to salicylic acid by hydrolysis.

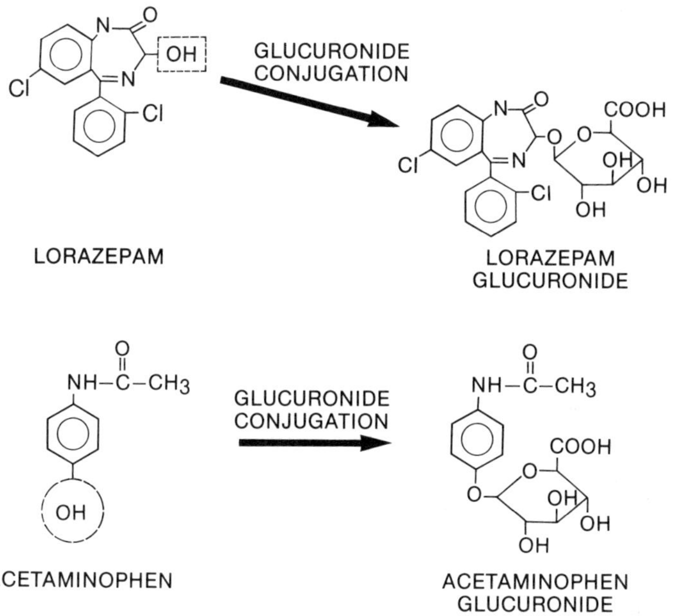

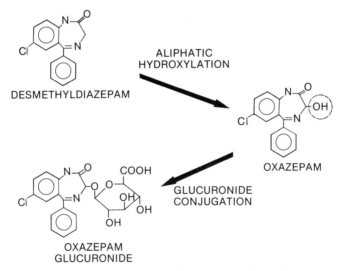

Figure 4–6. Examples of glucuronide conjugation reactions. *A,* Transformation of lorazepam to lorazepam glucuronide. *B,* Transformation of acetaminophen to acetaminophen glucuronide.

Figure 4–7. An example of sequential Phase I and Phase II biotransformation reactions. Desmethyldiazepam is initially biotransformed by the Phase I reaction of aliphatic hydroxylation, yielding the pharmacologically active product oxazepam. Oxazepam is then transformed by the Phase II reaction of glucuronide conjugation, yielding the pharmacologically inactive metabolite oxazepam glucuronide.

Table 4–3. PARTIAL LIST OF DRUGS THAT UNDERGO ACETYLATION IN HUMANS

Clonazepam
Hydralazine
Isoniazid
Nitrazepam
Phenelzine
Procainamide
Sulfanilamide

acid. Compounds already possessing a suitably located hydroxyl group (such as oxazepam, lorazepam, temazepam, acetaminophen, and morphine) require no Phase I transformation prior to glucuronide conjugation (Figure 4–6). Others require a Phase I hydroxylation prior to glucuronidation (Figure 4–7). Glucuronide and sulfate conjugates almost always are pharmacologically inactive and are readily excreted in the urine. It is of interest that elimination of some endogenous substances, such as bilirubin and certain steroid hormones, also involves glucuronide formation.

Acetylation is another important Phase II reaction (Table 4–3). This transformation involves attachment of an acetyl group to an amino substituent on the drug molecule. The amino group might be part of the intact parent compound (as with procainamide) or might be formed by a prior Phase I reaction (as with clonazepam and nitrazepam) (Figure 4–8). Metabolic products formed by acetylation often are pharmacologically inactive, but some acetyl conjugates are active. One important example is the acetylated product of procainamide (see Figure 4–8).

Humans can be tested to determine their capacity for drug acetylation. This is done by administration of a test or marker compound (such as sulfadimidine or isoniazid), which is biotransformed mainly by acetylation, followed by measurement of the rate and extent of metabolite formation. Results of such tests tend to cluster the population into groups of "slow" and "rapid" acetylators. This clustering effect is due to a genetically transmitted trait called the "acetylator phenotype." Most individuals are rapid acetylators, and the usually recommended dosage regimens for drugs in Table 4–3 are generally designed for this group. It must be remembered that slow acetylators might be much more sensitive to drugs in this category.

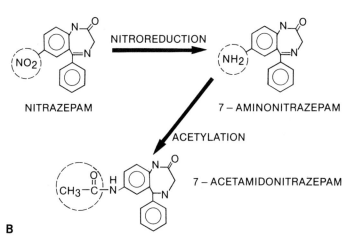

Figure 4–8. Example of acetylation reactions. A, Transformation of procainamide to the pharmacologically *active* metabolite N-acetylprocainamide. B, Sequential biotransformation of nitrazepam. The initial step is the Phase I reaction of nitroreduction, yielding 7-aminonitrazepam. This is followed by the Phase II reaction of acetylation, yielding 7-acetamidonitrazepam. Neither 7-aminonitrazepam nor 7-acetamidonitrazepam has significant pharmacologic activity.

SEQUENTIAL BIOTRANSFORMATION

Pathways of drug metabolism may involve many steps with many intermediate products (Figure 4–9; see also Figures 4–7 and 4–8). The intermediate products may be pharmacologically active or inactive. In some cases a biotransformation reaction transforms an inactive parent compound into an active metabolite. Clinical implications of active metabolites are discussed in Chapter 10.

FACTORS INFLUENCING PHASE I VERSUS PHASE II REACTIONS

What value is the knowledge about whether a drug is biotransformed by a Phase I as opposed to a Phase II reaction (Table 4–4)? Over the past decade considerable basic and clinical research has been done to evaluate the mechanisms controlling the activity of drug-metabolizing enzymes in humans. Most of these studies have focused on the Phase I oxidative reactions of hydroxylation and dealkylation and on the Phase II reaction of glucuronide conjugation. Intensive study of these particular pathways is appropriate, since they account for the biotransformation of the majority of drugs used in clinical practice.

Although both oxidation and conjugation reactions are carried out by hepatocytes, they are mediated by very different enzyme systems whose respective activities are controlled by different mechanisms. A given person's capacity for drug oxidation is quite consistent for most if not all drugs that are biotransformed by oxidative pathways.

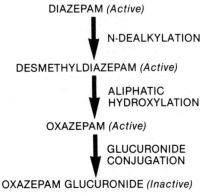

Figure 4–9. Examples of a sequential biotransformation pathway having both Phase I and Phase II components and metabolic products that are both active and inactive (see Figures 4–2 and 4–7 for the structures of each compound).

Table 4–4. SUMMARY OF PATHWAYS OF HEPATIC BIOTRANSFORMATIONS

Phase I (Preparative)
Hydroxylation
Dealkylation
Sulfoxidation
Nitroreduction
Hydrolysis

Phase II (Synthetic)
Glucuronide conjugation
Sulfate conjugation
Acetylation

That is, a given individual who is a fast or slow oxidizer of one drug is very likely to be a correspondingly fast or slow oxidizer of most or all drugs biotransformed by oxidation. Similarly, a person's capacity for conjugation is consistent from drug to drug metabolized by conjugation. On the other hand, an individual's capacity for oxidation generally is unrelated to his or her conjugating activity.

The differential control of drug oxidation and conjugation also is evident from studies of physiologic factors, disease states, and drug interactions that can alter drug-metabolizing capacity. Table 1–2 is a general list of factors known to alter drug metabolism. Those most extensively studied in the context of drug oxidation versus conjugation include old age, liver disease (hepatitis or cirrhosis), and coadministration of other medications (such as cimetidine, estrogens, isoniazid, or disulfiram) known to be metabolic inhibitors. All of these factors have a significant influence on the capacity for drug oxidation, causing a reduction in oxidative activity. However, the same factors have much less, if any, influence on the capacity for conjugation (Table 4–5). The clinical implications of impaired drug oxidation are most important during chronic dosage of drugs; this is discussed in Chapters 8 and 9. Drug interactions are discussed in more detail in Chapter 14.

Table 4–5. FACTORS INFLUENCING DRUG OXIDATION VERSUS CONJUGATION

	Influence on	
Factor	Phase I Oxidation	Phase II Glucuronide Conjugation
Old age	Impaired	Unchanged or slightly impaired
Liver disease (cirrhosis, hepatitis)	Impaired	Unchanged or slightly impaired
Metabolic Inhibitors	Impaired	Unchanged or slightly impaired

Table 4–6. PARTIAL LIST OF DRUGS THAT UNDERGO SIGNIFICANT RENAL
EXCRETION IN HUMANS

Amantadine
Aminoglycoside antibiotics
Cimetidine
Digoxin
Furosemide
Lithium
Nitrofurantoin
Ouabain
Penicillin antibiotics
Phenobarbital
Procainamide
Quinidine
Sulfonamides
Tetracycline

The Kidney

The kidney excretes water-soluble, polar metabolites of drugs formed by hepatic biotransformation. In the case of drugs that undergo glucuronidation (such as acetaminophen or lorazepam), more than 75 per cent of a dose may be recovered in the urine in the form of a glucuronide conjugate. There is also a relatively small but significant number of drugs that are excreted in the urine as intact compounds (Table 4–6). You will note that some of the drugs in this table have also been discussed as agents that undergo biotransformation. Quinidine and procainamide are examples of two antiarrhythmic drugs that are compounds having a "mixed" elimination pathway, being excreted partially intact and partially biotransformed to metabolic products.

Other Routes of Drugs Elimination

Together, the liver and kidney comprise by far the major mechanisms of drug elimination. Other routes are much less important. Very few drugs are excreted intact in the feces, unless their absorption from the gastrointestinal tract was poor to begin with. Volatile general anesthetics are both administered and eliminated by the lungs, but very few other compounds are excreted by this route. Even for those compounds whose odor we have come to recognize (paraldehyde, ethanol), elimination by the lungs accounts for only a small fraction of total drug clearance. Other routes of drug removal, such as excretion in sweat, tears, saliva, or breast milk, seldom are quantitatively important.

5

Intravenous Injection of Drugs

Only when a drug is injected directly into the vascular system is it certain how much drug reaches the systemic circulation and exactly how fast it gets there. Other routes of drug administration may be as reliable as intravascular injection, but this cannot be assumed unless proven by a pharmacokinetic study. Understanding drug behavior following intravascular injection is of considerable importance to clinicians, since drug disposition following other routes of administration is more easily understood if the kinetics of intravascular dosage have been elucidated. Strictly speaking, intravascular drug injection refers to both intra-arterial and intravenous dosage. In clinical practice, however, intravenous injection is by far the most common.

Rapid Intravenous Injection:
The Two-Compartment Model

Drug Behavior With Time

The one-compartment pharmacokinetic model assumes that the body consists of a single homogeneous space and that a drug injected directly into the vascular compartment is instantaneously distributed throughout the entire body (see Chapter 2). Despite the simplicity of this model, it is not applicable to the behavior of most drugs. The majority of exogenous compounds, when administered by rapid intravenous injection, behave as if the body consisted of at least two compartments. The two-compartment model is a surprisingly useful and widely applicable model of drug behavior.

Figure 5–1 is a schematic plasma concentration curve for a hypothetical drug following rapid intravenous injection ("bolus" injection) into a living organism. For purposes of clarity and for the reasons discussed in Chapter 3, the vertical concentration axis is logarithmic. Several points along the plasma concentration curve are labeled by Roman numerals. Interpretation of drug behavior at these particular points is shown schematically in Figure 5–2.

Point I represents that point in time at which the intravenous injection has just been completed. The density of drug molecules in the central or plasma compartment is at its maximum value. Since it is this compartment from which we measure drug concentrations, the plasma concentration curve therefore is at its maximum value of C_o. Drug distribution and elimination from the central compartment have just begun to take place, but neither process has yet occurred to any significant extent. At Point II, the distribution process is taking place. Note that the pipe connecting central and peripheral compartments has no "valves," indicating that drug molecules can pass in both directions. However, the "exit" or "elimination" pipe leading out of the central compartment has a one-way valve, since this represents the routes of irreversible drug elimination (see Chapter 4). As the distribution phase is taking place, the drug density in the central compartment, and hence the plasma drug concentration, is falling rapidly. Although elimination is in fact taking place during this phase, the rapid fall in drug concentration is due mainly to drug distribution out of the central compartment rather than irreversible drug elimination. Note that during the distribution phase, the density of drug in the peripheral compartment is lower than that in the central com-

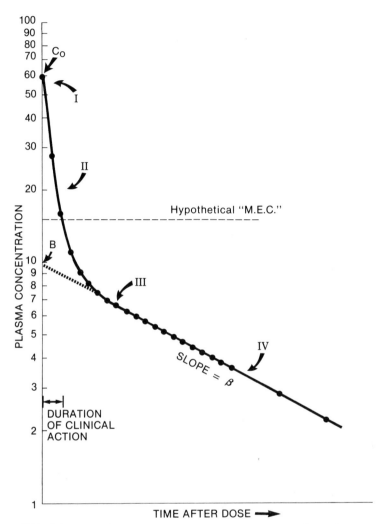

Figure 5–1. Schematic plasma concentration curve, using a semilogarithmic concentration axis, following rapid intravenous injection of a hypothetical drug. C_o is the peak concentration in plasma (or in the "central compartment") reached just at the end of the injection. B is the zero-time intercept of the elimination phase of the plasma concentration curve when extrapolated back to time zero. I, II, III, and IV represent the four stages of the plasma concentration curve as explained in the text and as indicated in greater detail in Figure 5–2. Note that the initial precipitous decline in plasma concentration between points I and III—attributable mainly to drug distribution—may be sufficient to terminate clinical activity if the plasma level falls below some "Minimum Effective Concentration" (M.E.C.).

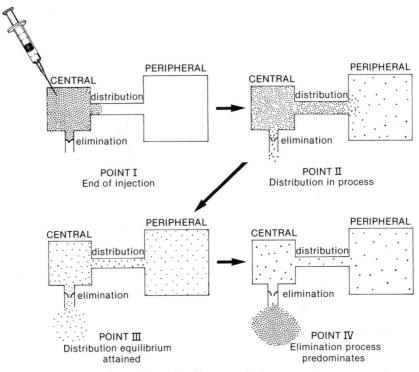

Figure 5–2. Four stages of drug distribution and elimination following rapid intravenous injection. Points I, II, III, and IV correspond to the points on the plasma concentration curve in Figure 5–1. *Point I:* The injection has just been completed, and drug density in the central compartment is highest. Drug distribution and elimination have just begun to take place, but neither has proceeded to any significant degree. *Point II:* Midway through the distribution process. The drug density in the central compartment is falling rapidly, mainly owing to rapid drug distribution out of the central compartment into the peripheral compartment. Note that the density of drug in the peripheral compartment has not yet reached that in the central compartment. *Point III:* Distribution equilibrium has been attained, and drug densities in the central and peripheral compartments are approximately equal. Drug distribution in both directions continues to take place, but the ratio of drug quantities in the central and peripheral compartments remains constant. At this point, the major determinant of drug disappearance from the central compartment becomes the elimination process, whereas previously drug disappearance was determined mainly by distribution. *Point IV:* During the elimination phase, the drug is being "drained" from both compartments out of the body (via the central compartment) at approximately the same rate.

partment; however, the peripheral compartment concentration is "catching up" with the central compartment concentration. Point III represents the time at which distribution equilibrium has been reached. At this point, the drug density in central and peripheral compartments is nearly identical. This does not mean that drug distribution is complete or terminated; in fact, drug distribution from central to peripheral compartments and back again continues to take place as long as any amount of drug is present in the body. Point III is, however, that point in time at which the ratio of drug amounts in central and peripheral compartments has reached a fixed number and will remain at that fixed ratio as long as the drug remains in the body. Note that at Point III in the concentration curve, the overall rate of drug elimination from the body appears to slow down. The plasma concentration curve is said to have entered the "elimination" phase, in which drug disappearance is mainly determined by irreversible elimination rather than distribution. Point IV represents some part of the elimination phase. Again, drug disappearance is determined mainly by elimination rather than distribution, although distribution to and from the central compartment obviously continues to take place. Note that as the drug is eliminated from the body via the central compartment, the drug density in both compartments declines in parallel.

Volumes of Distribution

Using the plasma concentration curve as observed in the clinical study, it is possible to calculate several importrant pharmacokinetic variables. Two such variables are the volumes of the mathematical compartments (see Chapter 2). The volume of the central compartment (V_c) is calculated as follows:

$$V_c = \frac{dose}{C_o} \hspace{5cm} 5.1$$

Several methods are available for calculation of the total apparent volume of distribution (V_d), which is the sum of the volumes of central and peripheral compartments. The most useful method provides a close approximation to V_d (but not the exact value) and is calculated by extrapolation of the elimination phase of the curve back to zero time intercept (Point B in Figure 5–1). Using this approximation, V_d is calculated as

$$V_d = \frac{dose}{B} \hspace{5cm} 5.2$$

Note that the approximation makes intuitive sense, since it uses an estimate of what the concentration would have been at time zero if we ignored the time necessary for distribution. As discussed in Chapter 2, these volumes of distribution are useful for conceptual purposes, but physiologic and anatomic interpretations should be done cautiously.

Half-Life of Elimination: Its Relation to Drug Action

The concept of half-life was described in Chapter 3. Drug half-life is perhaps the most commonly discussed pharmacokinetic characteristic, but the implications of half-life unfortunately are often misinterpreted.

A drug's half-life of elimination ($t\frac{1}{2}$ or $t\frac{1}{2}\beta$) can be calculated from the slope (β) of the plasma concentration curve during the elimination phase (Point IV in Figure 5–1) using the following relationship:

$$t\frac{1}{2}\beta \ = \ \frac{\ln 2}{\beta} \ = \ \frac{0.693}{\beta} \qquad\qquad 5.3$$

While the calculation of half-life is straightforward, its interpretation is more problematic. It is commonly assumed that the duration of clinical action of a drug after a single dose is related to its half-life; that is, long half-life implies long duration of action, whereas short half-life means short duration of action. Unfortunately this assumption is usually incorrect, because of how elimination half-life is defined for the two-compartment model. Half-life of elimination only describes the rate of drug disappearance *after distribution equilibrium is attained* but does not describe the rate or extent of drug distribution. In fact, distribution is a far more important determinant of the duration of clinical drug activity after single doses than is elimination half-life.

For most drugs (but not all), the molecular receptor site mediating clinical activity (see Chapter 1) behaves functionally as if it were a component of some central compartment tissue. For this reason the time-course of drug action after single doses often parallels the drug concentration in plasma. Clinical activity will be evident for as long as plasma concentrations remain above some "minimum effective concentration" (M.E.C., see Figure 5–1). When levels fall below the M.E.C., action is terminated. In Figure 5–2, the initial sharp decline in plasma concentrations during the early phase of drug distribution is sufficient to bring levels below the M.E.C., thereby terminating drug action. Drug elimination proceeds at a slower rate thereafter but is unrelated to the duration of clinical action. Physicians should take care to remember this dilemma—drug distribution is usually a more important determinant of drug action after single doses than is the rate of elimination.

Clearance

A final important concept is clearance. The term is probably most familiar as it applies to estimation of renal function. Creatinine clearance, for example, has dimensions of volume per unit time and is equal to the apparent volume of blood from which the endogenous product of muscle turnover, creatinine, is completely eliminated per unit of time. A creatinine clearance of 100 milliliters per minute indicates that 100 millimeters of blood or plasma are completely cleared of creatinine for each minute that passes. Higher values of creatinine clearance indicate more efficient removal of creatinine and hence more effective renal function; conversely, low values of creatinine clearance indicate that the overall efficiency of creatinine removal is lower, presumably owing to impairment of function of the eliminating organ. The overall efficiency of drug removal from the body likewise can be characterized by clearance, again having dimensions of volume per unit time. High values of clearance indicate efficient and generally rapid drug removal, whereas low clearance values indicate slow and less efficient drug removal. In general, the clearance of any given drug cannot exceed the total amount of blood flow to the organ responsible for clearance. In the case of a drug eliminated by hepatic biotransformation, the limiting factor in drug clearance would be hepatic blood flow, and drug clearance therefore could not exceed hepatic blood flow. Clearance can be calculated based on the plasma concentration curve, using the slope of the elimination of the curve (β) and the apparent volume of distribution (V_d) as follows:

Clearance $= \beta \times V_d$ 5.4

Note that any given value of clearance does not by itself tell you the exact values of half-life or volume of distribution. Rather, it is related to both of these factors. Clearance is an exceedingly important concept in pharmacokinetics. It is the single most important index of a given organism's capacity to remove a particular foreign chemical. Clearance furthermore is the major determinant of the extent of drug accumulation during multiple-dose therapy (see Chapter 8).

Biologic Versus Mathematical Relationships

Equation 5.4 indicates how clearance can be *calculated* once V_d and β have been determined but does not correctly indicate how the three variables are *biologically* related. In fact, V_d and clearance are biologically *independent* of each other, and Equation 5.4 is more properly rearranged as follows:

$$t\frac{1}{2}\beta = \frac{0.693 \times V_d}{\text{Clearance}} \qquad\qquad 5.5$$

The two factors on the right side of the equation are biologically distinct and unrelated variables. V_d is determined mainly by the physicochemical properties of the particular drug (such as water and lipid solubility, degree of ionization, and molecular size), the size and habitus of the organism to which it is administered, and the patterns of blood flow to various tissues. Clearance, on the other hand, is an index of the capacity for drug removal by the clearing organ or organs and is unrelated to V_d. On the left side of the equation is $t\frac{1}{2}\beta$, which is *biologically dependent on both V_d and clearance.* For a given drug in a given organism, $t\frac{1}{2}\beta$ would become larger or smaller in direct proportion to V_d if V_d were changed and clearance remained fixed. Similarly, $t\frac{1}{2}\beta$ would change inversely with clearance if V_d remained fixed. Simultaneous proportional changes in both V_d and clearance would leave $t\frac{1}{2}\beta$ unchanged. Because of the biologic relation of $t\frac{1}{2}\beta$ to *both* V_d and clearance, $t\frac{1}{2}\beta$ can be misleading when used as the sole index of drug metabolizing capacity.

Intravenous Infusion of Drugs

In many clinical situations it may be desirable to administer a drug by intravenous injection, since this is the most precise and reliable mode of drug administration. However, rapid intravenous injection generally leads to high initial drug concentrations in the plasma (central compartment), as indicated at Point I in Figure 5–1. For drugs with very narrow therapeutic indexes (such as lidocaine, quinidine, phenytoin, etc.), these high initial concentrations may often be associated with untoward drug effects. The hazards of excessively

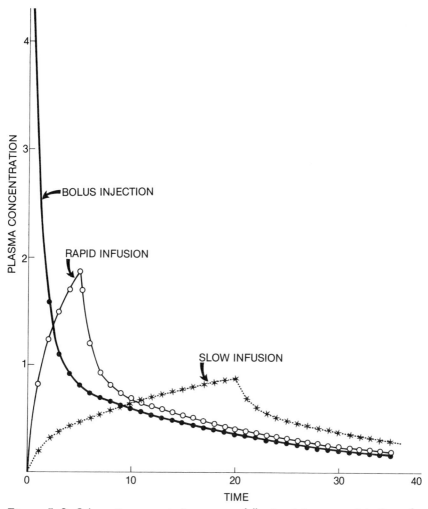

Figure 5–3. Schematic concentration curves following intravenous injection of a given drug dose at three different rates. After a rapid intravenous bolus injection, very high initial plasma levels are attained. The high peak level can be "blunted" or "smoothed out" by administration of the same dose in a slow intravenous infusion. Note that the blunting effect becomes greater as the infusion rate becomes slower.

high initial drug concentrations may be avoided without sacrificing the benefits of intravenous injection by using slow intravenous infusion rather than rapid injection. By this technique, the dose is administered by constant-rate infusion over a given period of time. Drug distribution takes place simultaneously with administration, thereby "blunting" the peak concentration and attenuating the apparent phase of drug distribution. The longer the infusion period, the lower the peak concentration achieved. Figure 5–3 shows plasma concentration curves following rapid injection of a given drug as compared with intravenous infusion at two different rates. Appropriate choice of dose and infusion rate can allow the benefits of intravenous injection to be preserved while simultaneously eliminating many of its hazards.

6

——

Oral Administration
of Drugs

Administration of drugs by the oral route is much more common than injection directly into the vascular system. However, a chain of events must precede the drug's reaching systemic circulation. The dosage form first travels from the oral cavity to the lumen of the stomach. Drugs already in liquid or solution form need not become further solubilized prior to absorption, but the more common solid dosage forms (tablets, capsules, or suspension) must enter solution in the normally acidic aqueous contents of the stomach. Simultaneously, the normal physiologic motility of the stomach begins to empty its contents into the duodenum and proximal small bowel, where most foreign chemicals are absorbed. Unless the drug has an unusually low molecular weight, it must traverse the membrane barriers lining the lumen of the proximal small bowel to reach the portal circulation. Only after traversing the hepatic vasculature do the drug molecules contained in portal blood ultimately reach the systemic venous circulation.

The bioavailability of an orally administered drug describes how fast and to what extent it reaches the systemic circulation after oral ingestion. Bioavailability depends upon the sequence of physiologic and pharmacologic processes described previously.

The Rate of Drug Absorption

Lag Time

When a drug is given by mouth it does not instantly begin to appear in the systemic circulation. The period of delay is termed the "lag time" (t_o) and is the time elapsing between drug ingestion and the beginning of its measurability in systemic circulation. A lag time prior to the start of the absorption is an almost universal phenomenon. First, the drug must traverse the distance between the mouth and the stomach, where the dosage form (unless it is already a solution) must disintegrate, enter solution, pass from the stomach to the absorptive site in the proximal small bowel, be absorbed into the portal blood, traverse the liver, and finally reach the systemic circulation. These processes are not instantaneous.

Lag times following oral drug administration usually range from 5 to 60 minutes, with the most common values falling between 10 and 30 minutes. Many factors can influence lag time, most of which also influence the rate at which the drug reaches the systemic circulation after it begins to appear (see below).

Absorption Half-Life

The meaning of exponential behavior and half-life was discussed in Chapter 3. Half-life characterizes the time necessary for any first-order process to proceed towards completion by another 50 per cent. In many cases, drug absorption, like drug elimination, is a first-order process. Instead of proceeding at a single, fixed rate, absorption takes place at continuously changing rates depending upon the amount of drug remaining to be absorbed. Shortly after absorption begins (i.e., after the lag time has passed), the rate of drug entry into the circulation is rapid, and the blood or serum drug concentration starts to rise (Figure 6–1). Simultaneously, distribution and elimination are taking place, causing removal of the drug from the blood. As more drug is

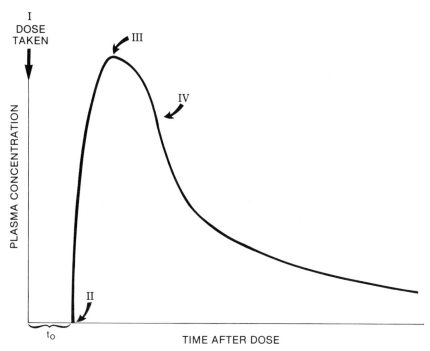

Figure 6–1. A typical plasma concentration curve following oral drug administration (the concentration axis is linear). At Point I, the dose is ingested. After the lag time (t_o) elapses, the drug begins to appear in the systemic circulation (Point II). Plasma concentrations rise until the rate of drug entry into blood equals the rate of removal by distribution and elimination, at which time the peak plasma level is reached (Point III). Thereafter, plasma concentrations fall (Point IV), since distribution and elimination are more rapid than absorption. Attainment of the peak concentration does not mean that the absorption process is complete, it continues, but at a continuously declining rate as the drug is removed from the gastrointestinal tract.

absorbed, the amount remaining to be absorbed is reduced, thereby continuously reducing the rate of entry. The peak blood or plasma concentration occurs when rates of drug entry (via absorption) and removal (via distribution and elimination) are equal. Thereafter, removal occurs more rapidly than entry, and the serum concentration falls, but absorption continues to occur *even after* the serum level reaches its peak.

When drug absorption is first-order, it can be characterized by an absorption half-life value ($t\frac{1}{2}a$) (Figure 6–2). As in the case of other first-order processes, short values of $t\frac{1}{2}a$ imply that absorption proceeds rapidly and peak concentrations in plasma are reached shortly after dosage. Larger values of $t\frac{1}{2}a$ conversely indicate slower drug absorption and a longer time between dosing and attainment of

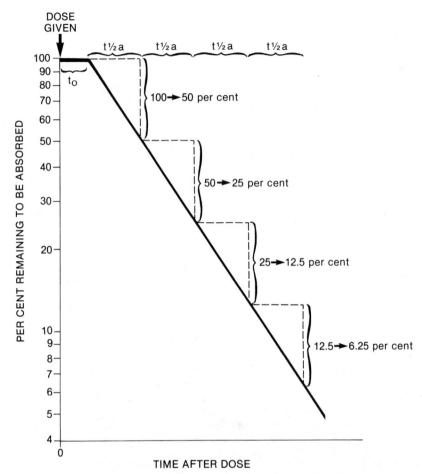

Figure 6–2. Semilogarithmic plot of the per cent of an orally administered dose remaining to be absorbed versus time since drug ingestion. After the dose is administered, the lag time (t_o) elapses before absorption begins. Thereafter, absorption proceeds as a first-order phenomenon. Each time an interval equal to the absorption half-life ($t\frac{1}{2}a$) elapses, the amount of drug remaining to be absorbed is reduced by another 50 per cent. After an interval of $4 \times t\frac{1}{2}a$, less than 10 per cent is remaining to be absorbed.

peak plasma levels. Consider a drug with an absorption half-life of 30 minutes. After a dose is given and the absorption process has begun, absorption will have reached 50 per cent of its final value in 30 minutes, 75 per cent in 1 hour, 87.5 per cent in 1.5 hours, and more than 90 per cent in 2 hours. As with other processes characterized by half-life values, first-order absorption has proceeded to more than 90 per cent of its final value after a period of at least $4 \times t\frac{1}{2}a$

has elapsed. Note that first-order drug absorption does not begin at the time of drug ingestion but only after the lag time has elapsed. Finally, it is important to realize that $t\frac{1}{2}a$ does not tell exactly *how much* of a given drug dose will eventually reach the systemic circulation. $t\frac{1}{2}a$ can be calculated and can be clinically useful, but the exact amount of the dose reaching the circulation may remain unknown.

A drug's absorption rate is a relatively "unstable" pharmacokinetic parameter. Even if the same individual ingests the same dose of the same drug under identical conditions on different occasions, the time and magnitude of the peak plasma concentration can vary considerably, and very different values of $t\frac{1}{2}a$ may be measured. Variability in $t\frac{1}{2}a$ generally is much greater than that observed in the elimination half-life $(t\frac{1}{2}\beta)$, which tends to be stable from time to time within the same individual. $t\frac{1}{2}a$ for a given drug is even more variable from person to person. In addition, $t\frac{1}{2}a$ is much more difficult to calculate in pharmacokinetic studies and has far less statistical reliability than does $t\frac{1}{2}\beta$.

Factors Influencing Drug Absorption Rate

Anything that can influence one or more of the links between drug ingestion and its appearance in the systemic circulation can influence lag time, $t\frac{1}{2}a$, and the time and magnitude of the peak plasma concentration. Such factors could involve the dosage form itself. Absorption rate could be slowed if a particular tablet preparation were tightly compressed or utilized very large drug particles, making it difficult for the drug to get into solution. Factors that reduce gastrointestinal motility and delay gastric emptying also can slow the rate of absorption. This can happen when a drug is taken on a full stomach or with an aluminum-containing antacid, or is coadministered with other agents (such as anticholinergics, tricyclic antidepressants, or opiates) that reduce gastrointestinal motility. Disease states that impair gastric emptying can also slow the rate of absorption. Conversely, absorption lag rate can be made more rapid if drugs are given in liquid rather than solid form or if patients are exposed to other drugs or disease states that stimulate gastrointestinal motility. In many cases, more than one such factor is present; when they operate in different directions, the net effect upon drug absorption may be impossible to predict.

Clinical Implications of Drug Absorption Rate

The lag time and $t\frac{1}{2}a$ collectively exert their greatest influence upon the early part of the plasma concentration curve. If t_o and $t\frac{1}{2}a$ are both short, then peak plasma concentrations are higher and reached earlier after an oral dose than if t_o and $t\frac{1}{2}a$ are long. The importance of the shape of the early part of the plasma concentration curve depends entirely upon the circumstances of drug ingestion. They are important when rapid onset of drug effects is desired: during the use of an oral analgesic (i.e., aspirin or acetaminophen) for the acute treatment of pain, the administration of a hypnotic agent to produce sleep, or treatment of a serious cardiac arrhythmia with an antiarrhythmic agent. In such cases, peak drug concentrations should be reached as soon as possible after the oral dose, and therefore the lag time and absorption half-life if possible should be small. Absorption rate may in fact be the major determinant of clinical drug efficacy, since slow absorption will delay and reduce peak plasma concentrations, which may not reach the minimum effective level (Figure 6–3).

In other clinical circumstances, the rate of drug absorption may be relatively unimportant. Such cases usually involve long-term drug therapy in which steady-state serum concentrations are much more important than peak levels attained after any given dose. Examples include the use of digitalis glycosides to treat congestive heart failure, tricyclic antidepressants to treat endogenous depression, or antituberculous chemotherapy. In some of these circumstances slow drug absorption is actually much more desirable than rapid drug absorption, since high peak levels produced by a given dose may produce transient side effects. This partly explains the use of "sustained-release" pharmaceutical preparations—dosage forms specifically designed to be absorbed slowly, thereby attenuating or eliminating the high peak concentrations observed after any given dose. Sustained-release preparations of quinidine, theophylline, diazepam, and other drugs are now available and widely used in clinical practice. It should be emphasized, however, that the actual clinical benefit of these sustained-release dosage forms, despite their theoretically sound rationale, has not always been conclusively demonstrated.

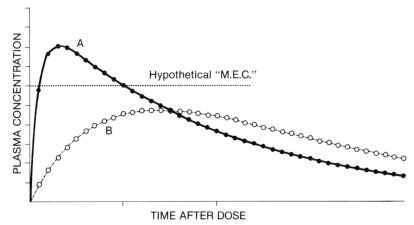

Figure 6–3. Schematic illustration of how absorption rate can influence the clinical effects of a drug in the acute dosage situation. In Case A, the absorption half-life is short, causing high peak plasma concentrations to be reached soon after the dose. The drug is clinically effective, since the minimum effective concentration (M.E.C.) is surpassed. In Case B, the size of the dose and the eventual completeness of absorption are *identical* to those in Case A. However, in Case B, the absorption half-life is 10 times longer. Because of slower absorption in Case B, the M.E.C. is never reached and the drug is clinically ineffective. Note that the plasma concentration axis is linear and that we have assumed for simplicity that the lag time is zero.

The Completeness of Drug Absorption

Drug absorption rate influences only the early part of the serum concentration curve and is important only in some clinical circumstances, but the completeness of drug absorption influences all parts of the serum concentration curve and is always of clinical importance. The completeness of drug absorption is sometimes called the "fractional absorption" (f) and describes that fraction of the administered dose that actually reaches the systemic circulation. The rate and completeness of drug absorption are theoretically distinct. It is true that many drugs that are slowly absorbed are also incompletely absorbed, but the two characteristics of drug absorption are best considered separately.

Measurement of plasma drug concentrations at multiple points in time after a given dose is usually sufficient to provide an estimate of t_o and $t\frac{1}{2}a$ for that particular trial. The completeness of drug absorption, however, cannot be determined from a single drug administration. The value of f for an orally administered drug in a given subject can only be determined from a two-part study. The first part involves intravenous drug administration to that subject; on another occasion, the drug, preferably the same dose, is administered orally. Multiple plasma concentrations determined after each dose are used to calculate the total area under the plasma concentration curve (Figure 6–4). The fractional absorption is calculated as the ratio of the total area under the curve after the oral dose (AUC_{oral}) to that measured after intravenous administration of the same dose (AUC_{IV}). Thus

$$f = \frac{AUC_{oral}}{AUC_{IV}} \qquad\qquad 6.1$$

Needless to say, enough time must elapse between the first and second trials for essentially complete drug elimination. An alternative method of determining f involves a study designed as described previously, except that urinary excretion (UE) of either the intact drug

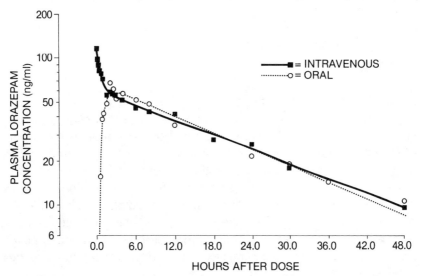

Figure 6–4. Example of a study of the completeness of absorption of oral lorazepam. A 4-milligram dose was given to a volunteer subject by intravenous infusion on one occasion and by mouth on another occasion. Multiple plasma concentrations were measured after each dose and the total area under the curve (AUC) determined by computer. The ratio of AUC_{oral} and AUC_{IV} was 0.94, indicating that absorption of the oral dose was 94 per cent complete in this particular study. (Note that the concentration axis is logarithmic.)

or a specific metabolite thereof is compared between the oral and intravenous administration trials. Thus

$$f = \frac{UE_{oral}}{UE_{IV}} \qquad\qquad 6.2$$

This approach is feasible, since urinary excretion is usually proportional to the amount of drug reaching the systemic circulation. Both methods for estimating f have advantages and disadvantages, and in some studies, both approaches are used simultaneously.

The importance of the completeness of drug absorption is being increasingly recognized. An orally administered drug may appear to be ineffective not because it is the wrong drug but simply because it is poorly absorbed from the gastrointestinal tract. Such situations cannot always be predicted without precise pharmacokinetic studies of drug bioavailability. Drugs with high fractional absorption tend to have relatively consistent values of f both within and between individuals. On the other hand, incompletely absorbed drugs can have variable and unpredictable absorption, both between individuals as well as from time to time within the same person. Accordingly, nearly complete absorption after oral administration is generally a desirable characteristic of an oral dosage form.

As with absorption rate, a number of factors can influence the completeness of absorption. Again, the dosage form is important. As a general rule, the completeness of drug absorption is greatest when administered in solution, followed successively by suspension, capsule, and tablet formulations; however, for well-absorbed drugs there may be little difference between the dosage forms. Coadministration of drugs with certain antacids or binding resins may impair the completeness of absorption, as may certain types of malabsorption syndromes. In general, the likelihood of complete drug absorption is enhanced when drugs are administered on an empty stomach.

The Need for Bioavailability Data

Clearly the bioavailability of orally administered drugs is an important determinant of their clinical action. Physicians should have as complete an understanding as possible about drug bioavailability as well as of those characteristics of his patients or the circumstances of drug administration that may influence bioavailability. Fortunately, the generation of reasonably precise data on drug absorption is becoming a requisite for the marketing of new agents. Whenever possible, physicians contemplating prescribing new pharmacologic agents should obtain and study such information.

7

Intramuscular Injection of Drugs

Clinicians commonly assume that intramuscular (IM) drug injection leads to rapid absorption of the drug into the systemic circulation, thereby assuring prompt and reliable onset of drug effects. IM injection is also thought to be safer than (and therefore generally preferable to) intravenous drug administration when parenteral dosage is required. These assumptions, along with the important practical consideration that IM injections but not intravenous infusions can be given by nurses, have led the IM route to become an exceedingly common mode of parenteral drug administration in clinical practice. An increasing number of studies, however, indicate that IM injection has important disadvantages and that the assumptions upon which its popularity is based are not always valid.

Factors Influencing the Rate of Absorption

As in the case of oral drug administration, absorption of drugs following IM injection depends upon a sequence of physicochemical and physiologic events. In many cases drug absorption from the site of injection proceeds as a first-order process and can be characterized by an absorption half-life ($t\frac{1}{2}a$). Small values of $t\frac{1}{2}a$ indicate rapid absorption, whereas larger values indicate slow absorption. Factors that can influence the absorption rate generally can be categorized as physicochemical or physiologic.

Physicochemical Factors: The Drug and Its Formulation

When a solution of a chemical is deposited in the interstitial space of muscle tissue, it can reach the interior of the vascular capillary network, and shortly thereafter the general systemic circulation, in two ways. Drugs that are very lipid-soluble ("lipophilic" drugs) readily and rapidly permeate the lipoidal membranes of capillary endothelial cells, thus making high lipid solubility a factor that favors rapid diffusion into capillaries. Water-soluble but lipid-insoluble drugs can diffuse from interstitial fluid to the capillary lumen only through the pores in the capillary membrane. Although these pores represent only a small fraction of the capillary surface area, the high rate of thermal motion of molecules in solution generally allows rapid diffusion of lipid-insoluble drugs into capillaries. Thus, a high degree of lipid solubility is not essential for rapid drug absorption following IM injection. On the other hand, some degree of water solubility is essential. The drug must be sufficiently water-soluble at physiologic pH to remain in solution long enough for absorption to occur. Drugs that are poorly water-soluble at physiologic pH may precipitate at the injection site and become unable to diffuse into capillaries (Figure 7–1). Precipitation at the injection site explains the very slow absorption of many drugs following IM injection (Figure 7–2). The most important of these are chlordiazepoxide, digoxin, phenytoin, quinidine, and a number of cephalosporin and penicillin antibiotics. Many other drugs have not yet been studied, and there is a clear need for rigorous pharmacokinetic assessment of the rate of absorption of all

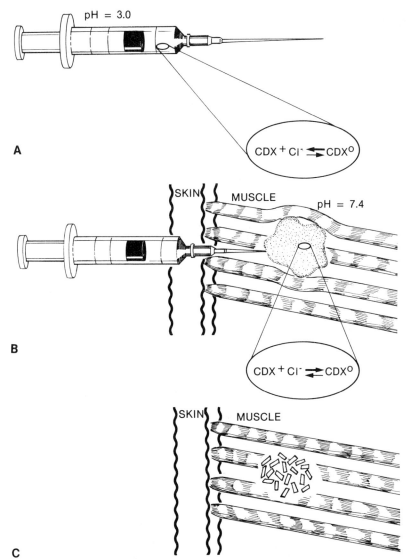

Figure 7–1. Sequence of physicochemical events following intramuscular injection of chlordiazepoxide.

Chlordiazepoxide is a weak organic base. In very acidic solutions, it exists mainly as the ionized, water-soluble, lipid-insoluble hydrochloride salt (CDX^+CL^-). In neutral or basic solutions, the water-insoluble, lipid-soluble un-ionized free base form (CDX^O) predominates.

A, The parenteral preparation of chlordiazepoxide is acidic, having a pH of about 3.0. As such, the water-soluble CDX^+Cl^- predominates (see schematic molecular enlargement) over CDX^O.

B, After injection into muscle tissue, the solution is quickly buffered to physiologic pH (about 7.4) by interstitial fluid. At this slightly alkaline pH value, equilibrium in the solution shifts dramatically, now favoring the water-insoluble free base (CDX^O).

C, Crystals of the free base precipitate at the injection site, causing absorption of the drug into the systemic circulation to proceed at the very slow rate determined by redissolution of the crystals. **55**

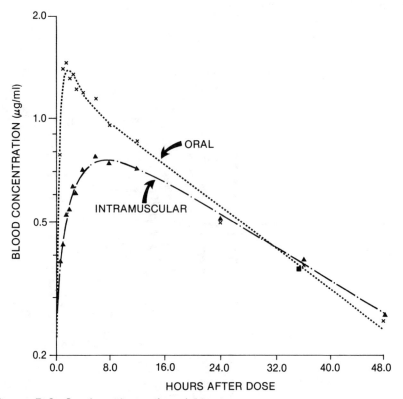

Figure 7–2. Semilogarithmic plot of blood concentrations of chlordiazepoxide following oral and intramuscular administration of 50 milligrams of chlordiazepoxide hydrochloride to 14 healthy subjects in a crossover study. Each point is the mean for all subjects at the corresponding time. Also shown are the pharmacokinetic functions. Note that the rate of absorption following intramuscular injection is much slower than that after oral administration of the same dose.

drugs given by IM injection. Until such data are available, clinicians should make no assumptions about the rate of drug absorption after IM injection.

Physiologic Factors

After a drug diffuses from the interstitial space into local capillaries, the rate at which it reaches the systemic circulation will be influenced by the blood flow to that muscle group. Blood flow at the injection site thus is a major determinant of absorption rates of drugs given by

IM injection. Blood flow per unit tissue weight is relatively high in deltoid muscles, intermediate in the vastus lateralis (thigh) muscle group, and low in the gluteal muscles. Pharmacokinetic studies have demonstrated that rates of drug absorption following IM injection into these three muscle groups are correspondingly rapid, intermediate, and slow. Needless to say, blood flow in fatty tissues is much less than that in muscles. Therefore, gluteal injections intended to be intramuscular, but which are in fact intra-adipose, certainly will be slowly absorbed. This commonly occurs with gluteal injections administered via short needles to female patients, particularly those who are obese. Since muscle blood flow increases with exercise, absorption rates generally are more rapid during exercise than at rest. Conversely, medical conditions that decrease blood flow to skeletal muscles (shock, hypotension, congestive heart failure, etc.) can dramatically slow the rate of drug absorption after IM injection.

Completeness of Drug Absorption

Complete precipitation of some drugs at the injection site can occur after administration in nonaqueous solutions or aqueous solutions at nonphysiologic pH. This probably explains most cases of incomplete bioavailability after IM injection. Precipitated particles can gradually redissolve and be absorbed by diffusion or can be removed by phagocytosis. However, both of these occur so slowly as to make absorption effectively incomplete.

Many of the drugs that are slowly absorbed after IM injection also are incompletely absorbed. Again, clinicians should make no assumptions about the completeness of drug absorption after IM injection until rigorous clinical pharmacokinetic data are available.

Adverse Effects of Intramuscular Injection

Fortunately, major complications of intramuscular drug injection appear to be infrequent. On the other hand, minor untoward effects, particularly local complications, probably are somewhat more common.

Local Complications

Adverse local effects of IM injection can be due to the mechanical aspects of the injection or to the properties of the drug or its solvent. Some degree of pain or local discomfort is probably inevitable. Pain is attributable to the mechanical trauma to the skin and underlying connective tissue by the needle. It can also be attributed to distention of the interstitial space within the muscle by the volume of fluid injected. Individual sensitivity to the painful effects of IM injection varies widely and unpredictably. Some individuals tolerate injections with essentially no pain and few if any complaints. Others describe excruciating pain, making the injection an exceedingly traumatic event, with severe anticipatory anxiety preceding each injection. Some measures can be taken to minimize pain. These include cleaning of the skin with a volatile spray such as ethyl chloride, use of a sharp, small-bore needle, and administration of the minimum possible total injection volume. Inasmuch as solutions of high tonicity and/or nonphysiologic pH can be extremely irritating and painful, solutions are best formulated in approximately isotonic aqueous solutions of neutral pH whenever possible. Unfortunately, the solubility characteristics of many drugs make this impossible.

Not surprisingly, IM injections also cause biochemical evidence of damage to muscle, as evidenced by elevations in circulating serum concentrations of creatine phosphokinase (CPK) derived from skeletal muscle. Release of CPK from damaged muscles is approximately proportional to the extent and severity of the damage. Consequently, elevations in serum CPK tend to be greatest when large volumes are injected into muscles, when the pH or tonicity of the injected solution is far from the physiologic range, or when the solution itself is intrinsically irritating. Although elevations in CPK by themselves are seldom if ever of consequence to a patient's health, they can confuse diagnoses of other diseases that are dependent upon measurement of serum CPK. The most notable of these is acute myocardial infarction. Although special techniques are now available that can differentiate CPK derived from skeletal as opposed to cardiac muscle, such techniques are not available in all hospitals. Thus, the clinical value of CPK in the diagnosis of acute myocardial infarction can be greatly compromised when such patients receive IM injections.

Pain and CPK elevations are annoying but generally transient local complications of IM injection. Irreversible sciatic nerve damage following gluteal injections is a widely publicized hazard, but this can be avoided if gluteal injections are always given in the upper outer quadrant. Skin pigmentation, intramuscular hemorrhage, septic or sterile abscesses, muscular fibrosis and contractions, and even gangrene have been reported following intramuscular injections, but these fortunately are very unusual.

Systemic Complications

Systemic or "total body" adverse reactions to IM injections can usually be attributed to the characteristics of the drug itself rather than the injection as such. The most ominous systemic reactions are anaphylactic responses and cardiovascular collapse. If such reactions develop shortly after an IM injection, they can be treated only by symptomatic measures, inasmuch as exposure to the offending agent cannot be terminated once the injection is completed. This points out one major disadvantage of IM as opposed to intravenous administration: if an untoward systemic complication develops during an intravenous infusion, the infusion can be immediately terminated, preventing further entry of drug into the body.

Slowly Absorbed Injections

As in the case of sustained-release oral preparations of drugs, formulations of drugs for IM injection may be deliberately formulated to produce a slow, "sustained" absorption pattern. This can be achieved by preparation of drugs in suspensions rather than solutions, by the use of viscous organic solvents such as glycerin or sesame oil, or by conjugating the active molecule to a long–chain fatty acid yielding an ester derivative that releases the active molecule slowly. Drugs commonly administered as slowly absorbed IM injections include benzathine penicillin, certain progestogens and androgens, and fluphenazine as enanthate or decanoate derivatives.

In specially selected circumstances this approach is quite rational and highly useful, inasmuch as the need for frequent drug administration is obviated and problems with patient noncompliance with oral drug regimens are reduced. On the other hand, the actual pattern of drug absorption following "depot" IM injections may be erratic and unpredictable, both between individuals and within the same individual from time to time.

Comment

Despite the popularity and convenience of IM drug injection, it is clear that this route of administration can be associated with major problems. The rate and completeness of drug absorption are by no means uniform and predictable. Furthermore, recipients of IM injections, particularly those who require many injections, will attest that the procedure often ranges from annoying to excruciatingly painful. Clinicians should carefully weigh the benefits and disadvantages of IM injection before this route of drug administration is chosen.

8

Chronic Dosage: The Extent of Drug Accumulation

The behavior of drugs following single intravenous, oral, or intramuscular doses can be extended to understand drug behavior during chronic therapy. This is of considerable importance, since the majority of drugs in clinical medicine are administered repeatedly rather than as a single, isolated dose.

Multiple-dose drug administration almost always leads to some degree of drug accumulation, unless doses are so widely spaced that the previous one is essentially completely eliminated before the next is given. The simplest model of drug accumulation involves continuous intravenous infusion, but this is clinically relevant only in unusual circumstances, as during infusion of drugs such as lidocaine, theophylline, nitroprusside, or heparin. More commonly, drugs are given as discrete doses repeated at specified times. After initiation of treatment with a fixed dose per unit time, drug accumulation proceeds until a "steady-state" is reached, after which no further accumulation occurs. At steady-state, the rate of drug entry into the body exactly equals the rate at which it is being removed by metabolism and excretion.

As long as drug elimination is "first-order" (see Chapter 3), multiple-dose therapy will always lead to attainment of a steady-state.

The following questions are pertinent to understanding drug behavior during chronic therapy: What is the extent of drug accumulation? That is, how much of the compound accumulates in the body and in the blood? How long does it take for steady-state to be attained? How much interdose fluctuation in blood levels is there once steady-state is attained? How does one approach the need for changing dosage or termination of therapy?

This chapter considers the question of the extent of drug accumulation. Other questions are considered in Chapter 9.

The Mean Steady-State Plasma Concentration

Unless a drug is given by continuous intravenous infusion, no single plasma concentration value characterizes the steady-state condition. This is because plasma levels fluctuate up and down over the dosage interval. Just after a particular dose, blood levels rise, reach a peak,

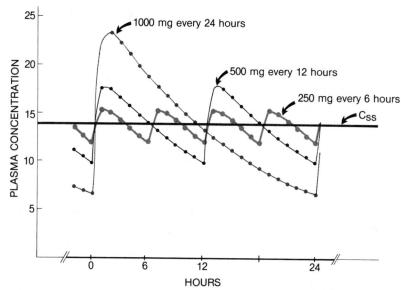

Figure 8–1. Plasma concentrations of a drug during chronic therapy using different dosage schedules. It is asssumed that $t\frac{1}{2}\beta$ is 12 hours and that treatment has gone on long enough for steady-state to be reached. Reducing or increasing both the size of the maintenance dose (D) and the interval between doses (T) changes the amount of interdose fluctuation in plasma levels but has no effect on the mean steady-state plasma level (C_{ss}), since C_{ss} depends on the *ratio* of D and T (see Equation 8.2).

then fall over the dosage interval until just before the next dose (Figure 8–1). The extent of the interdose fluctuation may be an important determinant of clinical response and depends largely on how frequently the daily dose is subdivided (see below). However, it is useful to consider a single value termed the "mean steady-state plasma concentration" (C_{ss}), which is related to the area under the plasma concentration curve over a dosage interval at steady-state (AUC_{ss}) and to the interval between doses (T) as follows:

$$C_{ss} = \frac{AUC_{ss}}{T} \qquad 8.1$$

This value is often quite useful in understanding multiple-dose drug therapy, although it contains no information on the extent of interdose fluctuation (see Figure 8–1).

Factors Influencing the Mean Steady-State Concentration

C_{ss} depends on the balance between drug entry and drug exit and can be calculated as follows:

$$C_{ss} = \frac{\text{Rate of drug entry into the body}}{\text{Total drug clearance}} = \frac{D/T}{\text{Clearance}} \qquad 8.2$$

where D is the maintenance dose given at a fixed dosage interval (T). It should be emphasized that D is not strictly the *administered* dose but rather the *absorbed* dose; that is, the dose that actually reaches the systemic circulation. This again brings up the important issue of the extent of drug absorption and bioavailability, considered in Chapters 6 and 7. However, for simplicity, we will assume that the administered dose is equal to the absorbed dose.

The determinants of C_{ss} can be categorized into those that are controlled by the physician (in the numerator) and those that are characteristics of that particular patient's capacity to eliminate that particular drug (clearance, in the denominator). Thus, the physician can alter C_{ss} by changing the dosage schedule. Increasing the size of the dose (D) or reducing the interval between doses (T) has the effect

Table 8–1. EFFECT OF CHANGES IN DOSE (D), DOSAGE INTERVAL (T), AND CLEARANCE ON MEAN STEADY-STATE PLASMA CONCENTRATIONS (C_{ss})

Change	Effect on C_{ss}
D increased	Increased
D decreased	Decreased
T increased	Decreased
T decreased	Increased
D and T both increased or decreased by the same factor	Unchanged
Clearance increased	Decreased
Clearance decreased	Increased

of increasing C_{ss}. Conversely, reducing D or prolonging T reduces C_{ss} (Table 8–1). Since clearance appears in the denominator, changes in clearance are inversely reflected in C_{ss}. Reduced clearance implies greater C_{ss}, whereas increased clearance reduces C_{ss}. Note also that a change in any one variable predicts an exactly proportional change in C_{ss}. For example, doubling the size of the maintenance dose exactly doubles C_{ss}; conversely, reducing the size of D by one-half also reduces C_{ss} by one-half. Changes in the two factors may offset each other. Doubling the dose and simultaneously doubling the interval between doses has no effect upon C_{ss}. For example, the value of C_{ss} for a dosage schedule of 250 milligrams every 6 hours should be identical to that for a dosage schedule of 500 milligrams given every 12 hours (see Figure 8–1).

The Accumulation Ratio

Equation 8.2 is useful in predicting the exact value of the mean steady-state concentration provided all the factors in the equation are known. Unfortunately, this is not always the case. Although D and T (i.e., the characteristics of the dosage schedule) are almost always known, an exact value of clearance may not be available. These limitations are partly obviated by use of the accumulation ratio (R_c). The use of R_c requires some assumptions; namely that a fixed maintenance dose (D) is given at equally spaced dosage intervals (T). Under these assumptions, R_c is defined as the ratio of the mean steady-state plasma concentration (C_{ss}) divided by the mean plasma concentration during the first T hours after the first dose (Figure 8–2). As such, it provides an estimate of the amount of drug present in plasma at steady-state in relation to that present during the first T hours after the dose.

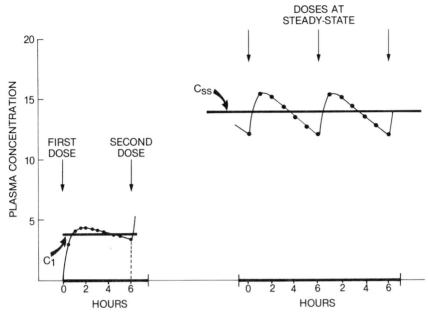

Figure 8–2. Example of how the accumulation ratio (R_c) is determined for a drug having an elimination half-life ($t\frac{1}{2}\beta$) of 12 hours, administered every 6 hours until steady-state is reached. The mean steady-state plasma concentration (C_{ss}), calculated from Equation 8.1, divided by the mean concentration during 6 hours after the first dose (C_1), gives R_c = 3.41. This can also be calculated using Table 8–1 or Equation 8.3. Since $t\frac{1}{2}\beta$ = 12 hours and T = 6 hours, the ratio of $T/t\frac{1}{2}\beta$ = 0.5, making R_c = 3.41.

R_c can be calculated based on knowledge of the interval between doses (T) and an estimation of the elimination half-life ($t\frac{1}{2}\beta$). Recalling that

$$\beta = \frac{\ln 2}{t\frac{1}{2}\beta} = \frac{0.693}{t\frac{1}{2}\beta} \qquad\qquad 3.2$$

R_c is given as

$$R_c = \frac{1}{1 - e^{-\beta T}} \qquad\qquad 8.3$$

Thus, the accumulation ratio depends upon the relation between the drug's elimination half-life and the interval between doses (Figure 8–3, Table 8–2). When the drug is administered at intervals exactly equal to its elimination half-life ($T = t\frac{1}{2}\beta$), the accumulation ratio is exactly 2.0, indicating that the mean steady-state plasma concentra-

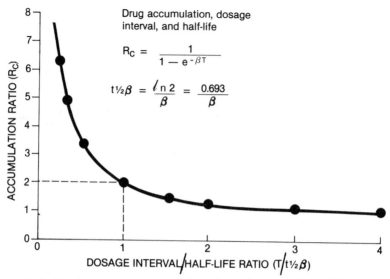

Figure 8–3. Graphic representation of the relation between R_c and the ratio of T and $t\frac{1}{2}\beta$. Note that when the dosage interval exactly equals the elimination half-life $(T = t\frac{1}{2}\beta)$, then $T/t\frac{1}{2}\beta = 1$ and $R_c = 2.0$.

tion is exactly twice the mean level after the first dose. When doses are given more frequently than the half-life (T less than $t\frac{1}{2}\beta$), greater accumulation is achieved. Conversely, when doses are less frequent than the half-life (T greater than $t\frac{1}{2}\beta$), accumulation is less extensive.

Calculation of R_c using Equation 8.3 can be of considerable value in clinical practice. An estimation of the elimination half-life is required, but knowledge of clearance is not. However, R_c does have limitations, inasmuch as it provides an estimate only of the extent of accumulation *relative* to the first dose. Equation 8.2 is necessary to estimate the *absolute* extent of accumulation.

Table 8–2. EXTENT OF DRUG ACCUMULATION IN RELATION TO ELIMINATION HALF-LIFE $(t\frac{1}{2}\beta)$ AND DOSAGE INTERVAL (T)

Ratio of Dosage Interval to Elimination Half-Life $(T/t\frac{1}{2}\beta)$	Accumulation Ratio (R_c)
0.25	6.29
0.33	4.89
0.5	3.41
1.0	2.00
1.5	1.55
2.0	1.33
3.0	1.14
4.0	1.07

Interdose Fluctuation

C_{ss} depends upon the *ratio* of the size of the dose and interval between doses (D/T). As long as both change by the sample multiple, C_{ss} does not change (see Table 8–1). However, such changes can have an important influence on the extent of interdose fluctuation, which is not reflected in C_{ss}. As one might suspect, increasing the interval between doses increases the extent of interdose fluctuation. When T is greatly prolonged, this leads to a more convenient dosage regimen, since doses need to be taken less frequently. However, the increase in convenience and greater likelihood of compliance are offset by an increase in the interdose fluctuation (see Figure 8–1). In some cases this may be excessive; that is, there may be periods during which the plasma concentration is too high, possibly leading to toxicity, followed by periods of subtherapeutic levels. Subdividing the daily dose into smaller increments administered more frequently reduces the extent of interdose fluctuation (see Figure 8–1). Although this is more desirable in therapeutic terms, it makes the dosage schedule inconvenient for the patient and thereby reduces the likelihood of proper compliance. In clinical practice, the final choice of a dosage schedule usually reflects a balance between the two objectives

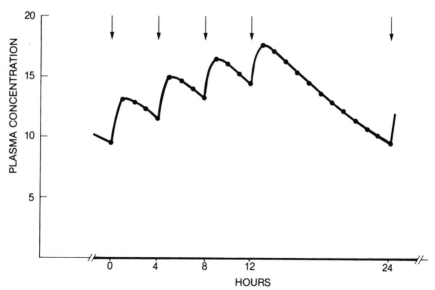

Figure 8–4. Plasma concentration curve for a drug given on a q.i.d. (e.g., 9 AM, 1 PM, 5 PM, 9 PM) dosage schedule. It is assumed that $t\frac{1}{2}\beta = 12$ hours and that therapy has proceeded long enough for steady-state to be reached.

of convenience of dosing and the need to minimize interdose fluctuation. For the majority of drugs, interdose fluctuation is acceptable when the dosage interval equals the elimination half-life ($T = t\frac{1}{2}\beta$). In this case, the accumulation ratio is equal to 2.0, and the plasma concentration in theory fluctuates by no more than 50 per cent above and below C_{ss}. This requirement still may impose constraints for many drugs. Procainamide, for example, has an elimination half-life of three hours; thus, dosing at intervals no less frequent than every three hours is generally necessary to achieve acceptable interdose fluctuation.

These considerations apply only to equally spaced dosage. The mathematical simplicity inherent in this assumption breaks down when doses are not equally spaced, as is common in clinical practice. Drugs that must be given in three or four daily doses, for example, are often given "t.i.d." or "q.i.d." rather than "every eight hours" or "every six hours." This yields a nonuniform plasma level pattern (Figure 8–4). The usual consequence is that plasma levels increase during the day, then fall during the night when no doses are given. The possible therapeutic implications of these dosage schedules should be carefully considered. In general, it cannot be assumed that a "q.i.d." dosage schedule is therapeutically equivalent to an "every six hours" schedule, even though the value of C_{ss} achieved by both approaches is the same.

9

——

Chronic Dosage: The Rate of Drug Accumulation

The extent of drug accumulation during multiple-dose therapy depends upon the size of each maintenance dose (D), the interval between doses (T), and the drug's total clearance (see Equation 8.2). In clinical practice, D and T are "known" quantities, but clearance is usually not known with certainty. Thus, precise prediction of the mean steady-state plasma concentration (C_{ss}) during multiple-dose therapy generally is not possible, and clinicians must settle for approximation of the extent of drug accumulation.

The second clinically important characteristic of multiple-dose therapy is the rate of drug accumulation; that is, the length of time following initiation of treatment that is required for the "steady-state" condition to be reached, after which there is no further drug accumulation. Estimation of accumulation rate is more straightforward and generally more accurate than prediction of the extent of accumulation. This is because the rate of accumulation depends almost entirely upon $t\frac{1}{2}\beta$ and is independent of D and T.

The Rate of Accumulation

Rates of drug accumulation during multiple-dose therapy and of drug elimination (either after a single dose or after the termination of multiple-dose treatment) are both determined by $t\frac{1}{2}\beta$. Accumulation is simply the inverse of elimination, and both processes occur with the same value of half-life. If one understands how the concept of half-life applies to drug elimination, understanding drug accumulation follows directly.

Consider a drug with an elimination half-life of $t\frac{1}{2}\beta$ administered as a fixed maintenance dose (D) at a fixed dosage interval (T). Each time an interval equal to $t\frac{1}{2}\beta$ elapses following the start of treatment, accumulation proceeds toward attainment of steady-state by another 50 per cent. That is, accumulation is 50 per cent complete after $1 \times t\frac{1}{2}\beta$, 75 per cent complete after $2 \times t\frac{1}{2}\beta$, and so on. Attainment of the steady-state condition is more than 90 per cent complete after an interval equal to at least $4 \times t\frac{1}{2}\beta$ has elapsed since the start of multiple-dose therapy (Figure 9–1). This is true *regardless* of the specific values of D and T; both of these quantities influence the *extent* of drug accumulation (see Equation 8.2), but they do not

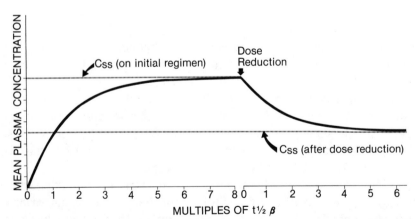

Figure 9–1. Simulated multiple-dose therapy with a hypothetical drug. Only mean plasma concentrations are shown, interdose fluctuation is not shown.

Treatment is initially started with a fixed dose per unit time. Note how the approach to the steady-state level (C_{ss}) is more than 90 per cent complete after $4 \times t\frac{1}{2}\beta$.

The dose per unit time is then reduced by exactly 50 per cent (arrow). The approach to the new steady-state proceeds similarly. The new C_{ss} is exactly half the former value.

influence the *rate* of accumulation. Regardless of what value C_{ss} is to be, the rate at which it is attained is always the same.

The same concept applies when either D or T is changed, thereby changing C_{ss}. Attainment of the new steady-state will also be more than 90 per cent complete after an interval equal to $4 \times t\frac{1}{2}\beta$ has elapsed since the change (see Figure 9–1).

Drug Accumulation: The Importance of $t\frac{1}{2}\beta$

$t\frac{1}{2}\beta$ is a major determinant of the rate of drug accumulation and of the *relative extent* of drug accumulation (R_c; see Chapter 8). A drug that is rapidly eliminated (short $t\frac{1}{2}\beta$) will rapidly attain the steady-state condition during multiple-dose therapy, and relative accumulation will be small (Table 9–1). Conversely, drugs that are slowly eliminated (long $t\frac{1}{2}\beta$) will accumulate slowly during multiple-dose therapy, and accumulation will be extensive (Figure 9–2). Thus, the potential for slow and "insidious" drug accumulation is greatest for those drugs that are most slowly eliminated. Bromide toxicity is a classic example. Symptoms of "bromism" develop slowly and are associated with long-term use of bromide-containing preparations. This is because $t\frac{1}{2}\beta$ for the bromide ion in humans is very long—approximately 12 days. Thus, accumulation will proceed at a correspondingly slow rate, and steady-state will be 90 per cent attained only after 48 days. Furthermore, accumulation will be very extensive. Assuming that the drug is given once daily, the accumulation ratio determined by Equation 8.3 will be 17.8.

Disease states that influence drug clearance have a profound effect on drug accumulation. These changes are readily predictable when the disease state *does not* change V_d, such that impaired clearance is inversely reflected by prolonged $t\frac{1}{2}\beta$ (see Equation 5.5). Assume that maintenance therapy with digoxin is initiated in a patient with normal renal function, for which $t\frac{1}{2}\beta$ is approximately 1.5 days.

Table 9–1. IMPLICATIONS OF $t\frac{1}{2}\beta$ DURING MULTIPLE-DOSE THERAPY

$t\frac{1}{2}\beta$	Rate of Accumulation	Extent of Accumulation
Long	Slow	Large
Short	Rapid	Small

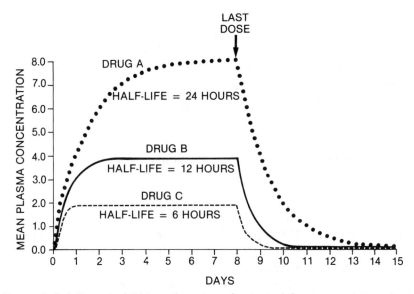

Figure 9–2. Influence of t½β on the rate and extent of drug accumulation. Again, only mean plasma concentrations are shown. It is assumed that the dose per unit time for all three drugs is the same and that they all have the same volume of distribution.

As t½β becomes shorter—going from Drug A to Drug C—the rate of accumulation becomes correspondingly more rapid and the extent of accumulation becomes less. The rate of drug "washout" after termination of therapy in each case is equivalent to the rate of accumulation.

The accumulation ratio is 2.7, and attainment of steady-state is essentially complete within one week (Figure 9–3). However, if the same individual had severe renal insufficiency, thereby prolonging t½β to approximately five days (assuming the same values of D, T, and V_d), accumulation occurs at a much slower rate, requiring three weeks to be more than 90 per cent complete. Furthermore, accumulation is much more extensive; the accumulation ratio is 7.7 (see Figure 9–3). This explains the well-recognized syndrome of slowly developing digoxin toxicity in patients with renal insufficiency and accounts for the recommendation that lower maintenance doses be used in such patients. A lower maintenance dose will lead to a correspondingly lower steady-state concentration but will not influence the rate at which steady-state is attained. Furthermore, even if the size of the maintenance dose is changed in such an individual, it will still require some three weeks for the new steady-state to be attained.

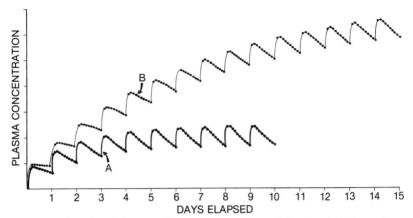

Figure 9–3. Simulated digoxin plasma concentrations following initiation of once-daily maintenance therapy with a fixed dosage. *A,* A patient with normal renal function; $t\frac{1}{2}\beta$ = 36 hours. *B,* A patient with severe renal insufficiency; $t\frac{1}{2}\beta$ = 5 days. Prolongation of $t\frac{1}{2}\beta$ increases the extent of accumulation and slows the rate of accumulation.

Loading Doses

The time required for attainment of steady-state following initiation of "maintenance" therapy may be unacceptably long. This problem arises most commonly in clinical situations requiring treatment with digitalis glycosides, antiarrhythmic agents, anticonvulsants, or certain antibiotics. In such cases, administration of a loading dose can eliminate or greatly reduce the time necessary to attain the steady-state condition (Figure 9–4). The decision as to whether a loading dose is needed is based upon assessment of clinical circumstances. However, choice of an appropriate loading dose should be based on pharmacokinetic principles. The accumulation ratio (R_c), calculated from Equation 8.3, is used to calculate the proper loading dose. Assuming that the maintenance dose and dose interval will be D and T, respectively, the loading dose (D_L) is

$$D_L = D \cdot R_c = \frac{D}{1 - e^{-\beta T}} \qquad 9.1$$

Thus, the loading dose depends on the dose and dosage interval that will be used during maintenance therapy as well as the elimination

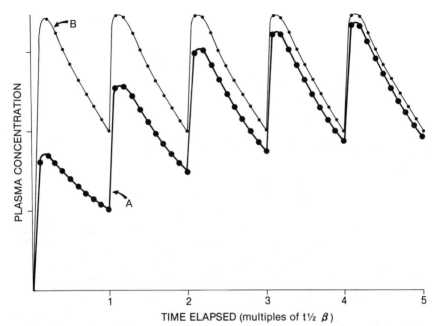

Figure 9–4. Simulated plasma concentrations for multiple-dose therapy initiated with or without a loading dose. A, Maintenance therapy is initiated with a fixed dose of a drug given at intervals to t½β, without a loading dose. B, Initiation of therapy with a loading dose equal to twice the maintenance dose, followed by maintenance therapy as above, leads to immediate attainment of the steady-state condition.

half-life of the drug (see Table 8–2). Consider, for example, the loading dose for a patient requiring digoxin therapy for which D = 0.25 milligram, T = 24 hours, and t½β = 36 hours. Using Equation 9.1, the appropriate loading dose is 2.7 times the maintenance dose, or 0.68 milligram.

Clinicians may not always remember the details of this scheme. However, a useful principle that can be easily remembered is that when the dosage interval is equal to the drug's elimination half-life, the loading dose is equal to twice the maintenance dose (see Figure 9–4).

10

——

Pharmacokinetic and Therapeutic Implications of Active Metabolites

Chapter 4 outlined the mechanisms by which the liver can modify or alter a foreign chemical to facilitate its removal from the body. It is increasingly recognized that the process of drug biotransformation does not necessarily lead to a loss of pharmacologic activity. In many cases, drug metabolites have essentially the same clinical activity as the parent compound (Table 10–1). These "active metabolites" almost always are the product of Phase I biotransformation reactions—oxidation, reduction, or hydrolysis. The Phase II reactions of glucuronide or sulfate conjugation usually do not lead to active metabolites, but acetyl conjugates sometimes are active, as in the case of the N-acetyl metabolite of procainamide. Biotransformation of drugs into active metabolic products complicates interpretation of pharmacokinetic data, because one must simultaneously consider the kinetic properties of both the parent compound as well as its active metabolites.

Table 10–1. PARTIAL LIST OF DRUGS WITH PHARMACOLOGICALLY ACTIVE
METABOLITES

Parent Drug	Active Metabolites
Acetohexamide	Hydroxyhexamide
Allopurinol	Alloxanthine
Amitriptyline	Nortriptyline
Amphetamine	Hydroxyamphetamine
Caffeine	Theophylline
Chloral hydrate*	Trichloroethanol
Chlordiazepoxide	Desmethylchlordiazepoxide
	Demoxepam
	Desmethyldiazepam
Clobazam	Desmethylclobazam
Clorazepate*	Desmethyldiazepam
Codeine	Morphine
Cortisone*	Cortisol
Diazepam	Desmethyldiazepam
Digitoxin	Digoxin
Flurazepam*	Desalkyl flurazepam
	Hydroxyethyl flurazepam
Glutethimide	4-hydroxyglutethimide
Halazepam	Desmethyldiazepam
Haloperidol	Dihydrohaloperidol
Imipramine	Desipramine
Lidocaine	MEGX, GX
Meperidine	Normeperidine
Mephobarbital	Phenobarbital
Methamphetamine	Amphetamine
Nitroprusside	Thiocyanate
Phenacetin	Acetaminophen
Phenylbutazone	Oxyphenbutazone
Prazepam*	Desmethyldiazepam
Prednisone*	Prednisolone
Primidone	Phenobarbital, PEMA
Procainamide	N-acetylprocainamide
Propranolol	4-hydroxypropranolol
Quinidine	3-hydroxyquinidine
Spironolactone*	Canrenone
	Canrenoate
Sulfasalazine	Sulfapyradine
Thioridazine	Mesoridazine
Trimethadione	Dimethadione

*Prodrugs (drug precursors).

Approaches to Clinical Use

Several issues must be kept in mind during the clinical use of drugs having one or more active metabolites. The rate and extent of metabolite accumulation are of major importance. After initiation of multiple-dose therapy with such drugs, metabolites accumulate either at the same rate or less rapidly than the parent compound, provided metabolite formation is a first-order process (see Chapters 3, 8, and 9). That is, the metabolite reaches its own steady-state level either at the same time or later than the parent compound (Figure 10–1). Conversely, after termination of chronic therapy, the half-life of disappearance of the metabolite is either equal to or longer than that of the parent compound, again provided metabolite formation is first-order. These constraints on the *rate* of accumulation do not apply to

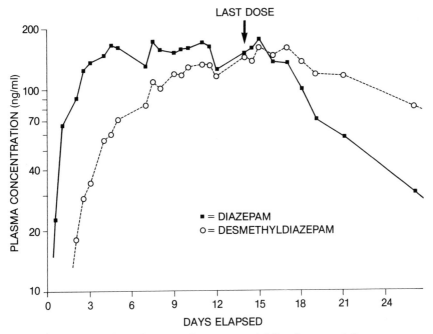

Figure 10–1. A healthy volunteer subject received 2.5 milligrams of diazepam every 12 hours for 15 days. Blood samples drawn just *prior* to each dose and at multiple points in time after the final dose were analyzed for concentrations of diazepam and its pharmacologically active metabolite desmethyldiazepam. Note that desmethyldiazepam accumulates more slowly than the parent compound. Once steady-state is reached, levels of both diazepam and desmethyldiazepam are nearly the same. After treatment is stopped ("last dose"), the relative rates of elimination parallel the rates of accumulation—desmethyldiazepam is eliminated more slowly than diazepam.

the *extent* of accumulation; the metabolite's steady-state level may be less than, the same as, or greater than that of the parent drug. For drugs having more than one active metabolite, the situation is obviously more complicated, but the same general principles apply as long as each metabolic product is formed by a first-order reaction.

Interpretation of serum concentrations of drugs with active metabolic products must involve consideration of all active compounds that are present. Frequently, clinical laboratories will provide quantitation only of the parent compound—this can be dangerously incomplete if active metabolites exist. Physicians who request serum drug concentrations for patients taking, for example, primidone, imipramine, or diazepam should *insist* that the laboratory provide simulta-

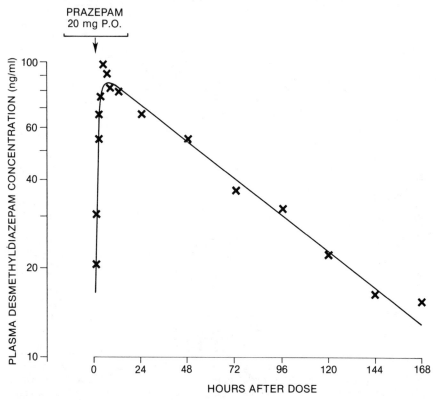

Figure 10–2. A healthy volunteer subject received a single 20-milligram oral dose of the benzodiazepine derivative prazepam. Multiple blood samples were drawn over the next seven days. Measureable amounts of intact prazepam were not present in blood at any time; desmethyldiazepam was the only active substance present. Thus, prazepam serves as a "prodrug" or precursor of desmethyldiazepam.

neous quantitation of phenobarbital, desipramine, or desmethyldiazepam, respectively. Only when serum levels of all active compounds are available can clinicians realistically expect that the laboratory results will provide information that is maximally useful in terms of understanding clinical effects. Unfortunately, reliable methods of quantitation of certain active drug metabolites (such as 4-hydroxypropranolol and 3-hydroxyquinidine) are not yet available for routine use in clinical laboratories. For this reason, knowledge of precisely how metabolites contribute to overall clinical activity may not always be complete.

Prodrugs

"Prodrugs," or drug precursors, in a sense are the exact opposite of drugs without active metabolites. For the latter group of drugs (such as oxazepam, lorazepam, acetaminophen, phenytoin, etc.), only the parent compound accounts for clinical activity—metabolic products are pharmacologically inactive. In the case of prodrugs, the parent compound either is pharmacologically inactive or reaches the systemic circulation only in very small or negligible amounts (Figure 10–2). Active metabolites account for essentially all of the clinical activity attributable to these drug precursors. Clinically important prodrugs are listed in Table 10–1. Clinicians should anticipate that requests for serum concentrations of such drugs should yield reports of "zero" except in unusual circumstances (such as acute overdosage).

11

Binding of Drugs to Serum or Plasma Proteins

Previous chapters have discussed serum or plasma drug concentrations as if the entire amount of drug present in the intravascular space were available to diffuse to extravascular sites of pharmacologic activity and biotransformation or excretion (such as liver or kidney). For a number of drugs used in clinical medicine this is not the case, since they are bound to protein constituents present in serum or plasma. Although drugs can bind to many proteins, albumin and alpha-one acid glycoprotein (AAG) are quantitatively the two most important proteins to which drugs can bind.

Nature of the Drug-Protein Interaction

Sites on a large protein molecule can attract and hold smaller drug molecules. The attachment is relatively loose and weak, unlike the strong covalent bonds that bind, for example, hydrogen and oxygen in the water molecule. The drug-protein interaction is reversible and dynamic—binding complexes are continuously being formed and broken. At equilibrium, the net rates of formation and breaking of the complexes (termed "association" and "dissociation") are the same, leading to constant relative concentrations of bound and unbound (free) drug. A simple characterization of the equilibrium condition is provided by the per cent or fraction of drug present in serum or plasma that is not bound to protein ("free fraction," or FF), defined as

$$FF = \frac{\text{Free (unbound) drug concentration}}{\text{Total (free plus bound) drug concentration}} = \frac{Cf}{Ct} \qquad 11.1$$

Since the sum of FF and the bound fraction (BF) must add to unity, then

$$BF = 1 - FF \qquad\qquad\qquad\qquad\qquad\qquad\qquad 11.2$$

Both FF and BF can range from 0.0 to 1.0 (0 to 100 per cent), depending on the extent of binding. It must be emphasized that FF, although clinically useful in many situations, does not provide specific or complete information on such factors as the number or type of binding sites on the protein molecule or the affinity or nature of the drug-protein interaction.

   To understand the implications of the binding of drugs to protein, it is of critical importance to distinguish free *fraction* and free *concentration*. In contrast to FF, the free or unbound concentration (Cf) is the absolute level (measured in units of amount/volume) of unbound drug in plasma. Cf is determined by the rate at which the drug reaches the systemic circulation and by the ability of the clearing organ to remove or convert the drug via biotransformation and/or excretion, as discussed in Chapter 4. This capacity for elimination of the unbound drug is called "unbound" or "free drug clearance" (see below). If a drug dose (D) is given repeatedly at regular time intervals (T) and if the entire dose reaches the systemic circulation (100 per cent bioavailability), then the average value of Cf at steady-state is expressed as

$$Cf = \frac{D/T}{\text{Unbound clearance}} \qquad\qquad\qquad\qquad 11.3$$

Note that Equation 11.3 is analogous to Equation 8.2, except that steady-state concentration of *free* drug replaces steady-state concentration of *total* drug and clearance of *free* drug replaces clearance of *total* drug. In fact, Equation 11.3 represents a refinement of Equation 8.2 that is appropriate for drugs that are extensively protein bound.

Note also that FF does not appear in Equation 11.3, indicating that Cf does not depend on the extent of protein binding. This is to be expected, since FF and Cf are determined by two different and independent physiologic processes. FF depends on the physicochemical interaction of the drug with protein, whereas CF depends on the balance between the rate at which the drug enters the body and the rate of elimination of unbound drug by biotransformation or excretion. Total concentration (Ct) simply "goes along for the ride," based on a rearrangement of Equation 11.1:

$$Ct = \frac{Cf}{FF} \qquad\qquad 11.4$$

Factors Influencing Protein Binding

Many factors can influence the extent of drug binding to protein. Two fundamental factors are the total drug concentration and the concentration of the binding protein. FF for many drugs remains relatively constant over a wide range of total concentrations, and a reduction of FF ("saturation of binding sites") is generally not observed unless total concentrations become so high as to be clinically irrelevant. However, changes in the binding protein concentration within the clinically relevant range can profoundly influence FF for many drugs. For albumin-bound drugs, reduction in serum albumin concentration can lead to an increase in FF, making disease states associated with hypoalbuminemia (such as cirrhosis, the nephrotic syndrome, severe malnutrition, etc.) important modulators of FF. Qualitative as well as quantitative changes in albumin can also influence FF. Renal disease and acute hepatitis, for example, can cause a reduced affinity of albumin for many drugs (leading to an increase in FF) even though the actual concentration of albumin in serum or plasma may be unchanged. For drugs bound to alpha-one acid glycoprotein, FF is quite sensitive to changes in AAG concentration (Table 11–1).

Table 11–1. PARTIAL LIST OF HIGHLY PROTEIN-BOUND DRUGS

Greater Than 90 Per Cent Bound (FF less than 0.1)	
Warfarin	Chlorpromazine*
Phenylbutazone	Oral hypoglycemics
Indomethacin	Furosemide
Propranolol*	Thiazide diuretics
Chlordiazepoxide	Ibuprofen
Oxazepam	Temazepam
Diazepam	
80 to 90 Per Cent Bound (FF between 0.1 and 0.2)	
Sulfisoxazole	Methadone*
Salicylic acid	Clofibrate
Digitoxin	Haloperidol*
Quinidine*	Lorazepam
Tricyclic antidepressants*	Phenytoin

*Drugs for which binding to AAG is quantitatively important.

Furthermore, the plasma concentration of AAG, unlike that of albumin which remains relatively constant, can vary widely in a given person. AAG is a "phase reactant" protein, and its concentrations increase greatly during acute severe illness (such as acute myocardial infarction, sepsis, injury, or shock) or during some chronic debilitating diseases (such as chronic infections or neoplastic disease). The increase in AAG concentrations can concurrently increase the extent of protein binding, and reduce FF, or drugs bound to AAG.

Other factors have been identified that may influence protein binding of drugs. In elderly individuals, there is a tendency for FF of drugs bound to albumin to increase, partly due to a reduction of serum albumin concentration that occurs with aging. FF of drugs can also increase owing to coadministration of other drugs that compete for binding sites. However, there still remain considerable differences in FF from person to person for most drugs. This individual variation usually cannot be explained by identifiable factors and remains poorly understood.

Implications of Protein Binding

The pharmacokinetic and clinical consequences of drug binding to albumin become increasingly important as FF becomes smaller, that is, for drugs that are very extensively albumin bound. When FF is very small (less than 0.1), apparently slight variations in FF can have important consequences (see Table 11–1). As FF becomes larger—in the range of 0.1 to 0.25—binding becomes somewhat less important. Values of FF greater than 0.25 generally imply that the consequences of protein binding are relatively unimportant.

Interpretation of Pharmacokinetic Data

Most pharmacokinetic studies base conclusions about drug disposition upon *total* rather than *unbound* serum or plasma concentrations. These conclusions may be misleading in the case of extensively protein-bound drugs. The smaller the value of FF, the greater the potential miscalculation. This problem arises because only the unbound fraction is available to diffuse out of the vascular system to sites of pharmacologic activity as well as to sites of biotransformation or elimination (Figure 11–1). When volume of distribution (V_d) is calculated from total drug concentrations (see Chapter 2), the extent of distribution of the *unbound* drug—the only fraction that is available for distribution—is underestimated to an extent that depends upon how small FF is. A more meaningful kinetic variable is the volume of distribution of the unbound or free drug (free V_d) calculated as

$$\text{free } V_d = \frac{V_d}{FF} \qquad\qquad 11.5$$

Similarly, clearance based on total drug concentrations (see Chapter 5) may be underestimated when FF is small, since for most (not all) drugs only the free drug can diffuse to organs responsible for clearance. Clearance of unbound drug, sometimes called "free clearance" is calculated as

$$\text{Free clearance} = \frac{\text{Clearance}}{FF} \qquad\qquad 11.6$$

It is important to note that under most circumstances, estimates of elimination half-life ($t\frac{1}{2}\beta$) will be the same whether based upon *total* or *unbound* drug concentrations, as long as FF does not vary as the total drug concentration changes.

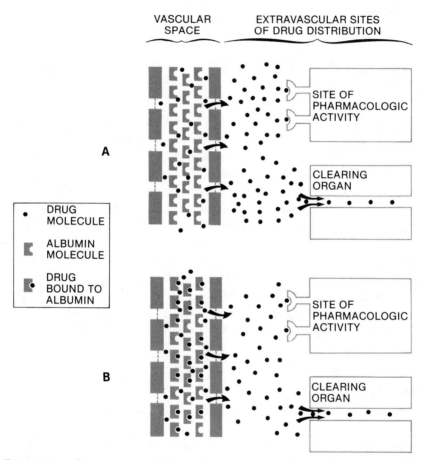

Figure 11–1. Effect of protein binding on pharmacokinetic calculations of clearance and volume of distribution.

A, A drug that is essentially unbound (FF $\cong$ 1.0). The entire amount of drug present in the vascular space is available for diffusion to extravascular tissues (such as the site of pharmacologic activity) and to the clearing organ responsible for drug elimination.

B, A drug that is extensively bound to albumin in the intravascular space. To deliver the same amount of drug to extravascular tissues—where albumin is not present—the vascular space must carry a much larger *total* (bound plus free) drug concentration, since only the unbound fraction can diffuse out of the vascular system. Calculation of V_d and clearance based upon *total* drug concentrations in serum or plasma underestimates the actual distribution and clearance of the unbound drug.

Interpretation of Serum Concentrations

Serum or plasma concentrations of drugs are commonly used to monitor therapeutic effects (see Chapter 13). It is generally recognized that serum level is more closely correlated with therapeutic efficacy or toxicity than is dose, because the concentration of drug in blood much more closely reflects the concentration at the site of pharmacologic activity. Unfortunately, most assay systems used to measure serum levels quantitate *total* (bound plus free) concentrations. The unbound concentration is of much more relevance than the total level, since only the unbound fraction can diffuse from the vascular system to the site of pharmacologic action. For highly protein-bound drugs, the actual extent of binding (that is, the actual value of FF) can have a great influence on the meaning of a total serum concentration in clinical practice. As FF becomes smaller, the potential clinical importance of binding becomes greater; a small difference in FF within one patient or between several patients implies that any given total drug level takes on a very different clinical meaning. This is discussed further in Chapter 13.

12

Nonlinear Pharmacokinetics

The properties of absorption, distribution, and elimination of most drugs used in clinical medicine are governed by first-order processes. Chapter 3 described in detail the characteristics of first-order processes, which can be summarized as follows: (1) they do not occur at a fixed rate, but rather proceed to completion at a rate that varies continuously over time; and (2) they are explained by an exponential function, which in turn can be used to calculate a characteristic number known as "half-life."

The therapeutic implications of first-order drug elimination are of considerable importance. When a first-order function governs drug removal from the body, then its elimination half-life remains the same regardless of the dose or the initial blood concentration. Large doses disappear with the same half-life as small doses. During multiple-dose therapy, the mean steady-state serum or plasma concentration is directly proportional to the dose (see Chapter 8). The steady-state level rises and falls exactly in parallel with the daily dose. The predictability of this relationship obviously simplifies the approach to titration of clinical response by adjustment of dosage.

For a few drugs, however, one or more processes governing drug disposition may deviate from those characterized as first-order. "Nonlinear kinetics" is a general term used to describe all such phenomena. Although such cases are exceptional, they involve some drugs that are widely used in clinical practice.

Saturable Metabolism

The most common type of nonlinearity encountered in clinical therapeutics is the case of saturable metabolism or biotransformation. The biochemical basis for this phenomenon lies in the hepatic enzyme system responsible for biotransformation of the drug. At relatively low doses or serum concentrations, drug-metabolizing enzymes function in a first-order manner such that the rate of drug elimination varies in proportion to concentration as follows:

$$\frac{\Delta C}{\Delta t} = -kC \qquad\qquad 12.1^*$$

As long as doses and serum concentrations remain in the relatively low "first-order" range, the drug has a half-life that is independent of dose (see Chapter 3) and mean steady-state serum concentrations are directly proportional to the daily dose (see Chapter 8).

However, as doses and serum concentrations get higher, the situation changes. Enzyme systems responsible for drug biotransformation become "saturated," and the rate of drug removal no longer increases at higher serum concentrations. In the range where enzyme activity is fully saturated, drug elimination is termed "zero-order," and proceeds at a fixed rate regardless of serum concentration as follows:

$$\frac{\Delta C}{\Delta t} = -V_{max} \qquad\qquad 12.2$$

---

*This is identical to Equation 3.1.

Table 12-1. DRUGS SUSPECTED OF HAVING SATURABLE METABOLIC PROCESSES AT CLINICALLY RELEVANT DOSES IN HUMANS

Aspirin (salicylate)
Ethyl alcohol
Phenytoin
Quinidine
Heparin
Tetracycline
Amobarbital

where V_{max} is the fixed rate of drug elimination expressed in units of concentration divided by time.

The implication of zero-order drug metabolism is that "half-life" is no longer an acceptable concept. During multiple-dose therapy, the steady-state serum concentration is *not* proportional to dose. Instead, a given increase in dosage will produce increments in serum concentration that are progressively greater as the total daily dose becomes greater.

Of several drugs suspected of having saturable metabolic processes (Table 12-1), phenytoin is among the most important because its kinetic profile changes from first-order to zero-order within the range of doses used clinically. The following case illustrates the type of problem that many physicians encounter. A patient diagnosed as having a seizure disorder is started on 200 milligrams per day of phenytoin. After two weeks of this regimen, a steady-state plasma concentration is measured and found to be 6 μg/ml—considerably below the usual therapeutic range of 10 to 20 μg/ml (Point A, Figure 12-1). The clinician accordingly adjusts the dosage to 300 milligrams per day. Two weeks later, the plasma concentration has risen to 9 μg/ml, still below the therapeutic range (Point B). The physician again raises the dose—to 400 milligrams per day, expecting the plasma level to rise proportionately to 12 μg/ml (Point C_1). Instead, the plasma concentration two weeks later is 26 μg/ml, and the patient has developed signs and symptoms of phenytoin toxicity (Point C_2). In this particular individual 300 milligrams per day is not enough and 400 milligrams per day is too much; the appropriate dosage falls somewhere in between, perhaps 300 milligrams alternating with 400 milligrams every other day.

Unfortunately, the point at which the saturation phenomenon becomes clinically important is not predictable from patient to patient, and phenytoin dosage adjustments must be made carefully and with frequent measurement of serum concentrations. The same can be said for other drugs, such as aspirin, with similar kinetic behavior.

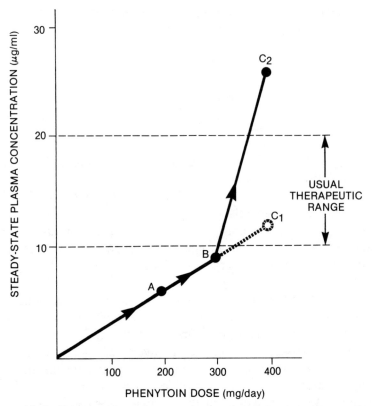

Figure 12–1. Relation of steady-state plasma phenytoin concentration to daily phenytoin dose. Increasing the dose from 200 to 300 milligrams per day (Point A to Point B) proportionately increases the plasma level. However, going from 300 to 400 milligrams per day does not produce the expected increase in plasma concentration (Point C_1), but rather a disproportionate increase (Point C_2). See text for further explanation.

Nonlinear Absorption

As in the case of drug elimination, a first-order, linear pattern of drug absorption from an extravascular site of administration has several important implications. First, the absorption process can be characterized by an absorption half-life ($t\frac{1}{2}a$) that is independent of dose. Second, the fraction of the dose absorbed into the systemic circulation also is independent of the size of the dose. As discussed in Chapter 6, variations within and between individuals in absorption kinetics can be quite large even for the same dose of the same drug. It may be difficult to determine whether this variation is a systematic

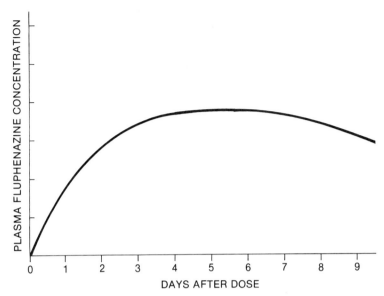

Figure 12–2. Schematic serum fluphenazine concentration curve following intramuscular injection at time zero of a "depot" preparation such as fluphenazine enanthate or decanoate. Note the nonlinear pattern of absorption (compare with Figure 6–1).

and replicable nonlinear or dose-dependent phenomenon or whether it is simply random variation.

Nonlinear absorption after intramuscular injection can occur because the drug is poorly water soluble at physiologic pH and precipitates at the injection site (see Chapter 7). A few substances, such as the antihypertensive drug guanethidine and the vitamin riboflavin, undergo nonlinear absorption due to their special physicochemical or pharmacologic properties. However, the majority of cases of nonlinear drug absorption result from deliberate pharmaceutical formulation of the compound to produce a "slow-absorption" or "sustained-release" pattern when given orally or by intramuscular injection. Procainamide, propranolol, theophylline, quinidine, and diazepam are examples of commonly used drugs that are available commercially in sustained-release oral dosage forms.

An extreme example of slow-release preparations are the "depot" injectable preparations of the antipsychotic drug fluphenazine. The drug is prepared as an ester derivative of either decanoic or enanthic acid, two long-chain fatty acids. The derivative is injected using a very viscous, oily solvent such as sesame oil. Before the active antipsychotic agent can reach the systemic circulation, the fatty acid ester derivative must be absorbed from the oily solvent, following which the ester is hydrolyzed by enzymes present in the blood. This process is very slow. Following a single intramuscular injection of one of these "depot" fluphenazine preparations, effective plasma fluphenazine concentrations can be maintained for days or even weeks, almost as if a continuous zero-order (constant rate) intravenous infusion were being given (Figure 12–2).

13

The Use of Serum or Plasma Drug Concentrations in Clinical Practice

The rationale for using serum or plasma drug concentration, rather than drug dosage, to monitor clinical response is theoretically sound. A sequence of events must take place before an orally administered drug reaches the site of pharmacologic action and thereby exerts a therapeutic effect (see Chapter 6). The drug must be absorbed from the gastrointestinal tract, pass through the liver (where biotransformation may begin), reach the systemic circulation, and become distributed to a variety of body tissues. Clinical response often depends entirely or in part on the drug concentration at the receptor site that mediates clinical action. Since the drug concentration in serum or plasma is closer to the site of action than is the orally administered dose, serum or plasma levels may correlate better with clinical response than with dosage. For this reason, plasma levels have attained increasing use as guides to therapeutics. Despite the value of this approach to therapeutic monitoring, recent evidence suggests a trend toward overuse and misuse of plasma drug concentration. Clinicians should recognize and understand those situations in which plasma levels may be of great value as well as those in which they may be of no value or even misleading.

When Plasma Drug Concentrations Are Clinically Useful

A number of requirements must be met before measurements of drug concentrations in plasma are clinically useful. These relate to the chemical characteristics of the drug, the nature of its pharmacologic action, and features of the underlying disease and its response to pharmacologic treatment. They can be summarized as follows:

1. The intensity of pharmacologic action must be proportional to the drug concentration at some receptor site of action.

This requirement makes intuitive sense. The intensity of the drug's pharmacologic action must rise and fall approximately in proportion to the rise and fall of its concentration at the receptor site of action.

2. The receptor site concentration must in turn be proportional to the unbound concentration of drug in plasma or serum.

As discussed in Chapter 11, the unbound drug fraction in plasma is available to diffuse out of the vascular system to sites of pharmacologic action. The plasma drug level cannot be useful unless there is free diffusion of the unbound drug to the site of action and the receptor concentration rises and falls in proportion to the unbound serum level.

3. The time-course of pharmacologic action must parallel that of drug concentration in plasma and at the receptor site.

Even if Requisites 1 and 2 are fulfilled, the serum level still would not be of value unless it reflected the intensity of pharmacologic action at the time that the level was measured.

These requirements are straightforward, but close examination indicates that they apply to relatively few drugs used in clinical practice. Table 13–1 gives approximate ranges of therapeutic plasma drug concentration for several representative drugs that have received considerable study. The ranges are not absolute; they are based on statistical analyses of clinical and pharmacokinetic studies and indicate the range of levels most likely to be associated with therapeutic response (see Figure 1–1).

Table 13-1. EFFECTIVE SERUM OR PLASMA CONCENTRATION RANGES FOR
REPRESENTATIVE DRUGS

Drug	Usual Range of Therapeutic Serum Concentrations	
Digitoxin	14–30	ng/ml
Digoxin	0.9–2	ng/ml
Phenytoin	10–20	μg/ml
Lidocaine	1.5–4	μg/ml
Lithium	0.5–1.3	mEq/liter
Nortriptyline	50–140	ng/ml
Procainamide	4–8	μg/ml
Quinidine	2–5	μg/ml
Salicylate	150–200	μg/ml
Theophylline	10–20	μg/ml

Factors Preventing Plasma Drug Levels from Being Clinically Useful

The following are examples of factors that can prevent fulfillment of the previously mentioned requisites and thereby reduce or eliminate the value of serum drug levels in clinical therapeutics.

Receptor Site Concentration not Proportional to Pharmacologic Effect

For some drugs either the intensity or time-course of pharmacologic action is not directly related to the receptor site concentration or to the concentration in plasma. Most notorious are the "hit and run" drugs that enter the body, cause a physiologic change, and then are completely eliminated before any clinical effect is observed. Such drugs include some ·of the anticancer agents and drugs that inhibit enzyme systems. The duration of drug exposure may also importantly influence the relation between clinical response and the receptor concentration. Adaptation or tolerance occurring during treatment with certain analgesics or central depressant drugs may reduce the intensity of pharmacologic action at any given drug concentration as time passes. Conversely, a particular plasma level may produce no therapeutic response early in the course of therapy, as in the case of tricyclic antidepressants.

Variations in Drug Distribution or Receptor Sensitivity

Characteristics of the patient or the underlying disease may alter either drug distribution from plasma to the various tissues or the sensitivity of the receptor site to any particular drug concentration. Such differences imply that the meaning of plasma concentrations would vary between different groups of patients or even from time to time within the same patient. The sensitivity of elderly individuals to many drugs is known to be increased, and this is explained at least in part by increased drug sensitivity at the level of the receptor. Thus, any given drug level might take on a different meaning in an elderly person as opposed to a young individual. Various disease states can also alter drug sensitivity and the interpretation of a given plasma level.

Drug distribution itself may also vary considerably as the result of disease states or patient characteristics. Distribution of medications within the body may vary considerably between men and women, suggesting that serum levels of some drugs may have to be interpreted differently between sexes. Diseases such as congestive heart failure or renal disease may alter characteristics of drug distribution between plasma and extravascular tissues and thereby alter the interpretation of plasma concentration.

Variations in Plasma Protein Binding

As discussed previously and in Chapter 11, only the unbound fraction of drug in serum or plasma is available to diffuse to sites of pharmacologic activity. Most laboratories use assay techniques that measure total (free plus bound) levels rather than the more pertinent unbound fraction. For drugs that are not extensively protein bound, this is probably not a clinically important limitation, since a low extent of binding implies that individual variations in binding have only a small impact on the total serum concentration. On the other hand, for drugs that are very extensively bound (see Chapter 11), small individual variations in binding can have a large impact on the meaning of the total plasma concentration. The greater the extent of binding, the smaller the proportion of total plasma level that is in the pharmacologically active, unbound form. All other things being equal, a total plasma phenytoin level of 20 μg/ml in a person with a free fraction of 5 per cent has the same meaning as a total level of 10 μg/ml in a person with a free fraction of 10 per cent (Figure 13–1).

Clinicians should be aware of those drugs that are extensively protein bound as well as those factors that may alter protein binding. In general, drug binding becomes less extensive (that is, the free fraction becomes higher) in the elderly, in those with low serum

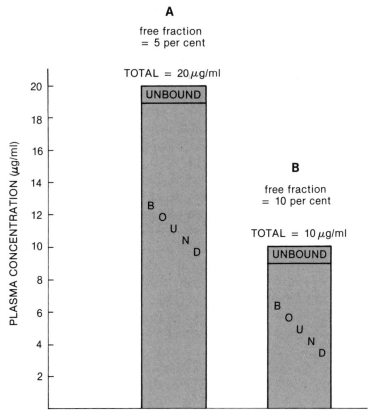

Figure 13–1. Example of how differences in protein binding can influence interpretation of plasma concentrations. Patients A and B are receiving the same daily dose of phenytoin, and it is assumed that both have the same unbound, or free, clearance of phenytoin. Based on Equation 11.3, both patients therefore have the same steady-state concentration of pharmacologically active free phenytoin. However, the *free fraction* of phenytoin is different (for whatever reason) between the two patients: 5 per cent in Patient A and 10 per cent in Patient B. Since total concentration depends on free concentration and free fraction (see Equation 11.4), total (free plus bound) concentration also is different between the two patients. All else being equal, an increase in free fraction leads to a decrease of total drug concentration without a change in free drug concentration and without a change in clinical activity.

albumin concentrations, in those with renal insufficiency, and in those taking other medications that may displace drugs from their binding sites on protein. The presence of these factors should alert the clinician to the possibility that the therapeutic and toxic total serum concentration ranges of the drug in question may shift downward.

Assay Technology

Implicit in the monitoring of serum drug concentration is the assumption that numbers provided by the laboratory are accurate. Most laboratories—particularly those affiliated with hospitals and academic institutions—have reasonably rigid standards of quality control such that the levels they provide can be considered as reasonably accurate. However, some assay techniques—particularly the immunochemical methods, such as radioimmunossay, radioreceptor assay, and enzyme multiplied immunoassay (EMIT)—may be subject to considerable inherent variability even in the best laboratories. The performance of outside commercial drug analysis laboratories often may be suspect. Some are as accurate and reliable as any academic laboratory, but others are concerned far more with financial gain than with analytic reliability. It is recommended that clinicians request quality-control data from such outside laboratories, particularly when they are relatively "unknown." Reliability should also be tested on a periodic basis using duplicate samples from the same patient or "spiked" samples containing known plasma concentrations.

As important as the reliability of the analytic technique itself is the question of what the technique is measuring. Some analytic procedures, particularly the older fluorometric or photometric methods but also the newer immunochemical methods, may quantitate not only the active drug present in plasma but also the levels of pharmacologically inactive metabolic products. Thus, plasma concentrations provided by such methods may overestimate the actual amount of pharmacologically active compound (Table 13–2). Conversely, analytic techniques may measure the concentration of parent compounds but may fail to quantitate the levels of important pharmacologically active metabolic products (see Chapter 10). Many drugs have active metabolites, and it is essential that serum concentration determinations for such agents quantitate not only the parent compound but also any active metabolites that may be present. Clinicians

Table 13–2. THE SPECIFICITY OF ASSAY METHODS FOR MEASURING PLASMA DRUG CONCENTRATIONS

Highly Specific ("The Gold Standard")
Gas chromatography—mass spectroscopy

Adequately Specific in Most Situations
Gas chromatography
Liquid chromatography ("HPLC")
Thin-layer chromatography

Questionably to Poorly Specific
Radioimmunoassay
Radioreceptor assay
Enzyme-multiplied immunoassay ("EMIT")
Spectrophotometry
Colorimetry

should take the initiative in attaining these objectives. Laboratories should be asked to specify the analytic techniques used for each drug measured. They should also state whether the technique is specific or nonspecific and whether active metabolites are simultaneously and/or separately quantitated.

Collection Technique

Even in the best of circumstances a plasma drug level can be rendered useless or even misleading if the timing or technique of sample collection is not properly planned. Of critical importance is the timing of the sample relative to the initiation of therapy and the dosage schedule.

After initiation of multiple-dose treatment with any drug, the time necessary for attainment of the steady-state condition depends on the drug's elimination half-life (see Chapter 9). After treatment has proceeded for four to five times the elimination half-life, the steady-state condition is more than 90 per cent attained. This is when a plasma drug concentration should be measured; if the plasma level is measured before steady-state has been reached, it will underestimate the actual steady-state level (see Figure 9–1). The same can be said when a plasma level is measured after a change in dosage. At least four to five half-lives must elapse before the new steady-state is reached (see Figure 9–1).

Clinicians frequently ignore the influence of interdose fluctuation

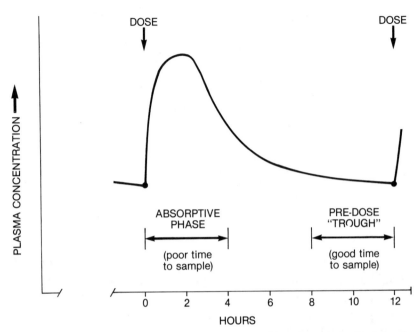

Figure 13–2. Schematic plasma concentration curve for a drug at steady-state when the dose interval is every 12 hours. Shortly after a dose, plasma levels rise, reach a peak, and then fall—this is the absorptive phase following that particular dose. This is a poor time to draw a blood sample for determination of plasma concentration, since it may be artefactually high. Although the duration of the absorptive phase cannot be predicted with certainty, a good estimate is up to four to six hours after each dose. The best time to draw a blood sample for measurement of plasma drug concentration is in the pre-dose, or "trough," period prior to the next dose.

on plasma drug concentrations. Unless a drug is given by continuous intravenous infusion, there is not a unique steady-state plasma concentration because the level rises and falls over each dose interval (see Figures 8–1 and 8–2). If the dosage interval is widely spaced for purposes of enhancing therapeutic compliance and convenience, the interdose fluctuation can be quite large (see Figure 8–1), such that the actual plasma level that is measured is strongly dependent on the time the sample is drawn relative to the most recent dose. If the blood sample is drawn within four hours of a dose, it is likely to coincide wth the "absorptive" phase and therefore be higher than the more representative "trough" level. In general, plasma concentrations measured just prior to a dose are the most useful, since clinicians can reasonably assume that levels are equal to or exceed this minimum or trough concentration (Figure 13–2). When the dosage schedule is irregular (see Figure 8–4), then even the pre-dose levels will vary throughout the day. Under these circumstances the concentration is most meaningful when measured just prior to the first dose of the day.

In some circumstances even the type of tube into which a sample is drawn can influence the measured plasma concentration. This is particularly true for drugs bound in part to alpha-one acid glycoprotein (see Table 11–1), since drug binding to AAG, and therefore total drug concentrations in plasma, can be altered by the plasticizers used to coat the rubber stoppers in certain brands of evacuated blood collection tubes (such as "Vacutainer"). Before a blood sample is drawn for measurement of a plasma concentration, clinicians should determine from the laboratory the type of tube to use; whether the sample needs to be refrigerated, handled urgently, or protected from light (owing to instability); and how it should be delivered to the analytic laboratory.

Comment

As with most technologic advances in clinical medicine, an initial period of enthusiasm is followed by an interlude of caution and critical reflection. We have now reached this point with the monitoring of serum or plasma drug concentrations. Critical appraisal of the value and nonvalue of such monitoring will ensure that the technique is used more wisely and cost-effectively.

14

—

Pharmacokinetic Drug Interactions: An Approach to the Clinical Problem

Additive clinical effects of drugs having similar pharmacologic properties have long been recognized. Simultaneous administration of alcohol and a barbiturate, for example, will produce greater central nervous system depression than when either is administered alone. Conversely, drugs having opposite pharmacologic actions may antagonize or cancel each other's actions. Administration of a stimulant drug such as caffeine, for example, is known to be an antidote to the depressant effects of alcohol.

Within the last two decades, a new category of drug interaction has become recognized. This is the pharmacokinetic drug interaction, in which two drugs having entirely different pharmacologic properties may potentiate or antagonize each other's effects. Pharmacokinetic interactions occur by several possible mechanisms that involve alteration of a drug's properties of absorption, distribution, elimination, or clearance.

The Historical Context of Drug Interactions

The relatively brief but highly visible history of pharmacokinetic drug interaction is in many ways typical of newly discovered scientific phenomena that can directly influence clinical medicine. Reports of clinically important interactions, particularly some that led to adverse consequences or even death in rare instances, began to appear in the late 1950s and early 1960s. These events were widely publicized and led to intense interest and attention from the scientific community. Studies of drug interactions increased in number, and a large number of interactions were discovered during the 1960s. The concern with the problem suggested to many that any two drugs administered simultaneously will interact to the detriment—and possibly even the death—of the individual unfortunate enough to be so mistreated. To say that a sort of drug interaction "hysteria" prevailed is probably not an exaggeration.

By the mid to late 1970s, scientists had critically re-evaluated the actual role of drug interactions in clinical practice. Based on the history of the drug interaction phenomenon and on evaluation of the mass of literature on the subject, most reasonable scientists reached the following conclusions:

1. Given the very high prevalence of polypharmacy—that is, coadministration of more than one drug to the same patient at the same time—actual drug interactions are unusual.

2. Even when pharmacokinetic drug interactions do occur, they are usually not of clinical importance.

3. Clinically important drug interactions are almost as likely to be beneficial to the patient as detrimental.

4. Of the very large number of review articles, books, and compendia devoted to the subject of drug interactions, the majority have inaccuracies and misinterpretations.

Sources of Information

One important source of data are studies involving in vitro systems or animal models. These studies usually are scientifically sound but not clinically relevant. Logic dictates that a drug interaction observed in a test tube or in a system not involving a living organism should not be assumed to occur in humans unless so proven. Animal studies do involve living systems but also may have little relevance to clinical therapeutics since they usually involve drug doses that are extremely large on a weight basis. Furthermore, the metabolic profile of most drugs in animal species differs substantially from that in humans. Many drug interaction studies involve rodents such as rats or mice, in which the metabolism of foreign chemicals differs greatly from that in humans. Again, logic dictates that interactions observed in animals do not necessarily apply to humans until so proven. Nonetheless, interactions reported from in vitro and animal studies have been widely perpetuated as clinical fact.

Data from human studies are more easily interpreted yet do not always give a true picture of clinical reality. Many drug interactions have been observed and described as isolated case reports or as small series of patients. A few of these have turned out to be of general clinical importance, but the majority prove to be spurious or coincidental events that are never replicated. Again, many such case reports have been misinterpreted and stated as general clinical fact.

Controlled clinical pharmacokinetic studies of drug interactions comprise a large proportion of the literature in this area. The experimental subjects usually are healthy volunteers. If drug y is suspected of producing a change in the kinetic profile of drug x, the volunteers are first administered one or more test doses of drug x in the control state to determine its kinetic profile without coadministration of drug y. In a second phase of the study, drug x is readministered to the volunteers, this time during or after exposure to drug y, the agent suspected of producing an interaction. Comparison of the kinetics of drug x in the two conditions allows conclusions about whether a drug interaction does exist and how large an interaction it is.

The scientific strength of these studies should not be underestimated, since they provide important information on the fate of foreign chemicals in humans. Yet formal pharmacokinetic studies do not always provide an estimate of whether interactions are of clinical importance. For example, the observation of an interaction (or of a noninteraction) in healthy young volunteers does not necessarily predict what will happen to the actual patient population for which the drugs were intended: patients who may be elderly and those with underlying disease states altering the metabolic profile and clinical response to drugs. Secondly, a statistically significant drug interaction in a pharmacokinetic study by no means implies a clinically important phenomenon. For example, if drug y produces a 10 per cent change in the clearance of drug x in all subjects who participate in the study, this will be highly significant in the statistical sense but unlikely to be of importance in clinical practice.

Interpreting the Literature: What to Look For

The quantity of literature on pharmacokinetic drug interactions is so large that no clinician or scientist can possibly expect to master or understand it all. Physicians who coadminister drugs in clinical practice must expect to make frequent trips to the library to locate and evaluate the original scientific data relevant to the particular clinical problem. The ability to evaluate this literature is an important clinical skill. The following approach is recommended:

1. Review articles, books, compendia, and other secondary sources on drug interactions should be viewed with skepticism and suspicion. With the exception of a few well-documented interactions whose clinical importance is established, clinicians should obtain information mainly if not exclusively from primary sources.

2. Data derived from in vitro studies, animal investigations, or isolated case reports in humans can be viewed as suggestive but by no means definitive. If such data are all that are available, the likelihood of a clinically important drug interaction should be regarded as not established.

3. Data from controlled clinical pharmacokinetic studies in humans should be evaluated critically. What is the magnitude of the interaction? Does it vary from subject to subject? What duration of exposure to drug y is necessary for the interaction to develop?

4. Data from pharmacokinetic or epidemiologic studies involving actual patients are probably the most helpful to the questioning clinician. In such realistic populations, how often does an interaction occur? How often does it alter decisions about drug therapy? Are there particular patients or groups of patients in whom the likelihood of interaction is increased?

Comment

The previous discussion is not intended to minimize the clinical problem of pharmacokinetic drug interactions but rather to place it in proper perspective. Authors of secondary sources generally are well-intentioned and are attempting to meet the need for compendia that bring together and summarize a vast amount of scientific information. Nonetheless, such sources invariably contain inaccuracies and misinterpretations, which unfortunately tend to be self-perpetuating. It is therefore essential that practicing physicians concerned about drug interactions develop the ability to locate and critically assess original scientific sources.

15

Pharmacokinetic Drug Interactions: Mechanisms of Drug Interaction

Many pharmacokinetic drug interactions have been discovered in the last two decades. Although relatively few are of clinical importance, the number is still too large for clinicians to learn them all. Understanding how to evaluate drug interaction literature (discussed in Chapter 14) is therefore an important clinical skill, as is conceptual understanding of the mechanisms of drug interaction. The following framework is a useful aid to understanding drug interaction mechanisms.

Interactions Involving Drug Absorption

The Rate of Drug Absorption

Interactions altering drug absorption rate are important only when absorption rate in itself is important. Slowing of absorption of an analgesic or a hypnotic could be of clinical importance, since attainment of rapid and high peak blood levels may be essential to produce clinical efficacy (see Figure 6–3). On the other hand, interactions changing the rate of absorption of antibiotics or digitalis glycosides quite likely are unimportant, since absorption rate is not a determinant of action of these drugs.

The rate of drug absorption is reduced by any influence that slows gastrointestinal motility. Administration of anticholinergic medications or opiate analgesics will reduce gastrointestinal motility and slow the absorption of almost any other medication given by mouth. Conversely, drugs such as metoclopramide that enhance motility may speed up absorption of other drugs. Probably the most common interaction involving drug absorption rate is due to the nonspecific effect of food in the stomach. Coadministration of drugs with meals rather than on an empty stomach will slow absorption of most medications, since a full stomach slowly empties its contents into drug absorption sites in the proximal small intestine. Antacids can have a variable effect on drug absorption rate, depending on the components of the particular preparation. Antacids containing large amounts of magnesium salts may speed the rate of drug absorption owing to the effect of magnesium on motility. Conversely, antacids containing predominantly aluminum salts will slow gastric emptying.

The Completeness of Drug Absorption

Interactions involving the completeness of drug absorption are more likely to be of clinical importance. Changing the rate of absorption often simultaneously changes the completeness of absorption, and the two mechanisms usually should be considered together.

Administration of tetracycline with iron salts, sodium bicarbonate, or certain antacids can greatly reduce tetracycline absorption owing to the formation of nonabsorbable complexes. Very few other drug interactions are this dramatic. Certain binding resins and surfactant products, such as cholestyramine or kaolin-pectin, may interfere with the absorption of other drugs (such as digitoxin or lincomycin), but these interactions are usually not dramatic and may be clinically unimportant. Coadministration of drugs with food has a variable and unpredictable effect. Food may increase, have no effect on, or decrease the completeness of drug absorption, depending on the constituents of the meal and the chemical properties of the drug.

The likelihood of drug interactions involving drug absorption can be minimized if drugs are always given on an empty stomach rather than with meals and if patients on multiple medications receive the drugs separately (i.e., separated in time by more than one-half hour) rather than together.

Interactions Involving Drug Distribution

Interactions having this mechanism are unusual. Administration of guanethidine with tricyclic antidepressants immediately and dramatically reduces the antihypertensive efficacy of guanethidine, because the antidepressant drug displaces guanethidine from its intracellular site of action. A second recently discovered interaction involves digoxin and quinidine. Coadministration of quinidine and digoxin reduces the extent of digoxin distribution, probably owing to a reduction of a digoxin uptake into skeletal muscle. The two drugs also interact by a second mechanism, in which quinidine impairs the renal clearance of digoxin.

A second type of distributional interaction involves protein binding displacement (see Chapter 11). Consider drug x, which is tightly bound to plasma protein, and recall that only the unbound fraction is pharmacologically active. If drug y has a greater affinity for protein than does drug x, coadministration of drug y will cause a displacement of drug x from its binding site, thereby transiently increasing its unbound plasma concentration (Figure 15–1). The increase in free drug levels may cause a transient increase in clinical activity until the increased free concentration undergoes metabolism and excretion. When a new equilibrium is established, the absolute unbound concentration and clinical activity of drug x are the same as they were before drug y was administered, but the total (free plus bound) concentration is lower (see Chapter 13). These interactions rarely are of clinical importance but may arise when two tightly bound drugs are coadministered.

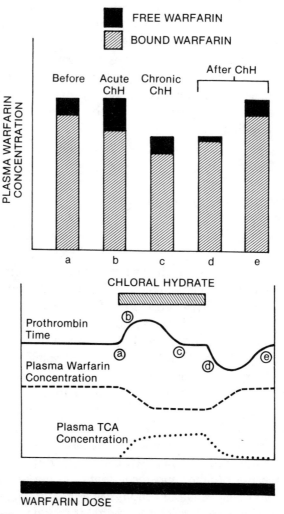

Figure 15–1. Effect of chloral hydrate administration on oral anticoagulant therapy (schematic). A patient on "stable" anticoagulant therapy, receiving a constant daily dose of warfarin, is started on chloral hydrate (ChH) because of insomnia (Point a, top and bottom). Trichloroacetic acid (TCA), the major metabolite of chloral hydrate, displaces warfarin from protein-binding sites, temporarily increasing the plasma concentration of unbound, pharmacologically active warfarin (Point b, top), thus potentiating its hypoprothrombinemic effect (Point b, bottom). Because the liver metabolizes the excess free warfarin, the effect is a transient one. During chronic chloral hydrate therapy (Point c, top and bottom), total (free plus bound) warfarin plasma concentrations are smaller than before chloral hydrate, but unbound warfarin concentrations as well as clinical anticoagulant effect are the same (see Chapters 11 and 13). When chloral hydrate is discontinued (Point d, top and bottom), the reverse happens—warfarin effect is transiently antagonized because unbound warfarin occupies the protein-binding sites previously taken up by TCA. Several days after chloral hydrate is stopped (Point e, top and bottom), the pre-chloral hydrate situation is re-established. Notice that the daily dose of warfarin was never changed.

Interactions Involving Drug Clearance

Stimulation of Hepatic Microsomal Function

Among the first drug interactions to be described were those involving stimulation of hepatic drug-metabolizing capacity, sometimes termed "enzyme induction." A number of drugs (Table 15–1) are known to stimulate the activity of enzyme systems responsible for the biotransformation of other drugs, causing an increased clearance and reduced steady-state plasma concentration of other coadministered drugs (see Equation 8.2). The most important and widely publicized of such interactions involves impairment of oral anticoagulant activity by coadministration of barbiturates (Figure 15–2). Barbiturates, as well as other drugs known to have enzyme-inducing properties, may stimulate the clearance of many other coadministered medications. However, such interactions will be of clinical importance only if the

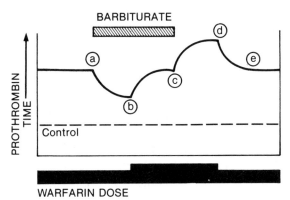

Figure 15–2. Effect of barbiturate administration on oral anticoagulant therapy (schematic). A patient on "stable" anticoagulant therapy, receiving a constant daily dose of warfarin, is started on a barbiturate hypnotic because of insomnia (Point a). Due to hepatic microsomal enzyme induction and increased clearance of warfarin due to the barbiturate, steady-state warfarin concentrations fall (see Equation 8.2), warfarin activity is antagonized, and prothrombin times fall toward control values. Increasing the daily warfarin dose (Point b) compensates for the increased clearance due to enzyme induction and restores plasma warfarin levels and prothrombin times to the previous therapeutic range. When barbiturate therapy is stopped, thus removing the enzyme-inducing stimulus (Point c), prothrombin times become excessively prolonged, possibly leading to hemorrhage unless the situation is corrected by a physician. Reducing warfarin dosage (Point d) to the pre-barbiturate level restores therapeutic anticoagulation (Point e).

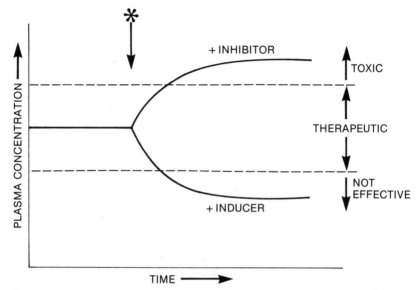

Figure 15–3. Consequences of a pharmacokinetic drug interaction for a drug having a narrow therapeutic index (such as in Figure 1–1, B). It is assumed that the drug is administered at a constant daily dose long enough for the steady-state to be reached, and the steady-state plasma concentration (C_{ss}) is assumed to be in the therapeutic range. At the vertical arrow with the asterisk (*) above, either an enzyme inducer or an enzyme inhibitor is co-administered. The inducer causes an increase in clearance, causing C_{ss} to fall (see Equation 8.2). Conversely, the inhibitor would cause a decrease in clearance, causing C_{ss} to rise. Since the therapeutic range of the drug is narrow, the interaction with the inhibitor would cause toxicity, and the interaction with the inducer would cause loss of effectiveness.

change in steady-state plasma concentration is sufficient to cause a change in clinical effect (Figures 15–3 and 15–4). It is important to recognize that interactions involving enzyme induction do not occur immediately after exposure to the inducing agent. Enzyme induction is a slow process; it can take anywhere from a few days to a few weeks to become clinically evident. Conversely, removal of the enzyme-inducing agent will lead to correspondingly slow disappearance of the induced state.

Impairment of Drug-Metabolizing Capacity

In contrast to the enzyme inducers, agents that impair or poison metabolic function exert their effect rapidly (see Table 15–1). For

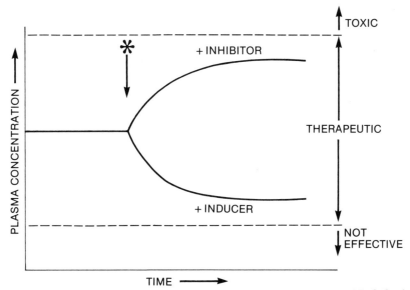

Figure 15–4. The identical pharmacokinetic situation as that in Figure 15–3. In this case, however, the therapeutic index of the drug in question is wide (such as in Figure 1–1, *A*). The same drug interactions and changes in C_{ss} as those in Figure 15–3 are of less clinical consequence this time, since the alteration in C_{ss} is not sufficient to cause toxicity or ineffectiveness.

example, coadministration of chloramphenicol to a patient already receiving an oral antidiabetic medication such as tolbutamide will cause an immediate increase in plasma tolbutamide concentration and increase the likelihood of hypoglycemia. You will note that ethyl alcohol appears in Table 15–1 as both an inducer and an inhibitor. This is because chronic alcoholism acts to stimulate hepatic microsomal function, whereas acute intoxication impairs metabolizing function. The net effect of acute alcohol ingestion by a chronic alcoholic is unpredictable.

As in the case of enzyme induction, an interaction involving enzyme inhibition cannot be assumed to be of clinical importance (see Figures 15–3 and 15–4).

Interactions Involving Renal Function

The list of drug interactions involving renal clearance of medications is relatively small, and such interactions may be therapeutically

Table 15–1. PARTIAL LIST OF DRUGS REPORTED TO STIMULATE OR IMPAIR
METABOLISM OF OTHER DRUGS

Drugs Reported to Stimulate Metabolism	
Barbiturates	Glutethimide
Carbamazepine	Phenytoin
Ethyl alcohol	Rifampin
Drugs Reported to Impair Metabolism	
Disulfiram	Ethyl alcohol
Isoniazid	Estrogens
Chloramphenicol	Methylphenidate
Tricyclic antidepressants	Cimetidine
Propoxyphene	Propranolol

beneficial as well as unfavorable. Probenecid is commonly administered to patients receiving penicillin antibiotics to delay the excretion of the penicillin and prolong its therapeutic effect. Probenecid has also been reported to alter renal excretion of other drugs such as cephalosporin antibiotics, aminosalicylic acid, nitrofurantoin, and isoniazid. Another renal interaction involves digoxin and quinidine, in which quinidine impairs the renal clearance of digoxin.

When Are Drug Interactions Likely to Be Important?

Polypharmacy is by no means a source of automatic danger. On the contrary, knowledgeable and careful coadministration of medications is far more likely to be therapeutically beneficial than harmful. The unusual instances in which clinically important drug interactions are possible can be either avoided or used for therapeutic benefit if physicians understand the possible mechanisms of interaction and the literature can be realistically evaluated.

Drug interactions are most likely to be clinically important when the magnitude of the interaction is very large or when the patient is seriously ill and is in a delicate therapeutic "balance." Of equal importance is the therapeutic index of the drug in question. Agents having a narrow boundary of therapeutic effectiveness—when the difference between lack of efficacy and toxicity is very small—are those most likely to be importantly influenced by coadministration of other drugs that may interact pharmacokinetically (see Figures 15–3 and 15–4).

APPENDIX

Sources of Pharmacokinetic Data

Our recommendations to clinicians regarding locating and evaluating pharmacokinetic data are similar to those we made for evaluating drug interactions. Whenever possible, consult primary sources. Many textbooks and review articles on clinical pharmacology and drug therapy are available, and most of these contain pharmacokinetic data. However, it is usually not possible to determine with certainty whether the data in these secondary sources are reliable and up-to-date. As in the case of data on drug interactions, misinformation on pharmacokinetics often is perpetuated from one review article or textbook chapter to the next. Unfortunately, the notoriously least accurate and most outdated pharmacokinetic information appears in the "approved" package inserts for individual drugs and in the *Physician's Desk Reference.*

One important exception to the most uncertain reliability of secondary sources is the journal *Clinical Pharmacokinetics,* published by the Australasian Drug Information Service. In addition to publishing original research data on drug disposition, this journal devotes much of its space to review articles on the pharmacokinetics of drugs in humans. Individual articles are written by researchers who have experience with the kinetic properties of the drug or drug class in question as well as with its clinical use. The articles comprehensively review the pertinent literature and present in readable tabular form the drug's properties in healthy humans as well as factors (such as old age, disease states, and drug interactions) that can alter the pharmacokinetic profile. Because articles in this journal are published promptly after acceptance, the material is up-to-date.

How to Find Pharmacokinetic Data

Clinicians looking for kinetic data on a drug or drug class may find a recent review article in *Clinical Pharmacokinetics* by scanning the index or table of contents of recent volumes. The next approach is

---

Table A–1. LITERATURE SOURCES FOR CLINICAL PHARMACOKINETICS

Reviews
Clinical Pharmacokinetics

Original Data: The Most Important Sources
Clinical Pharmacology and Therapeutics
Clinical Pharmacokinetics
Journal of Clinical Pharmacology
British Journal of Clinical Pharmacology
European Journal of Clinical Pharmacology

More Sources of Original Data
Journal of Pharmacokinetics and Biopharmaceutics
Biopharmaceutics and Drug Disposition
Drug Metabolism and Disposition
Drug Metabolism Reviews
International Journal of Pharmaceutics
International Journal of Clinical Pharmacology
Journal of Pharmaceutical Sciences
Journal of Clinical Psychopharmacology
Pharmacology
Journal of Pharmacology and Experimental Therapeutics
Arzneimittel-Forschung
Clinical Pharmacy
Therapeutic Drug Monitoring
Psychopharmacology
Acta Pharmacologica et Toxicologica
Drugs
Drug Development Research
Journal of Pharmacy and Pharmacology

to scan the appropriate topic heading in *Index Medicus,* which collects and catalogues esentially every article published in the biomedical periodical literature. *Index Medicus* is published monthly, then collected into a single yearly edition at the end of each year. Within 30 to 60 minutes, the titles of all publications on a drug or drug category during the last five years can be reasonably completely reviewed, and clinicians can then locate actual publications reporting pharmacokinetic data.

The journals most likely to carry such articles are listed in Table A–1. The most familiar is *Clinical Pharmacology and Therapeutics,* which is available in most hospital libraries. The others in the primary list can be found in libraries of larger medical centers and medical schools.

Original data on drug disposition in humans also appear in a number of other scientific journals whose primary focus is not specifically clinical pharmacology or pharmacokinetics. Occasionally articles of particular importance are published in the widely circulated general clinical journals (*New England Journal of Medicine, Annals of Internal Medicine, Journal of the American Medical Association, Archives of Internal Medicine, American Journal of Medicine, Lancet, British Medical Journal,* etc.) or in clinical subspecialty journals.

Index

Note: Page numbers in *italics* refer to illustrations; page numbers followed by (t) refer to tables.

Acetylation, in hepatic biotransformation, 28, 28t, *29*

Biotransformation, hepatic, acetylation in, 28, 28t, *29*
  and elimination of drugs, 22–24, *23*, 24t, *25*, 26, *26*, *27*, 28, 28t, *29*, *30*, 30–31, 31t. See also *Drug(s), elimination of.*
  dealkylation in, 24, 24t, *25*
  drug interactions and, *115*, 115–116, *116*, *117*, 118t
  glucuronide conjugation reactions in, 26, *27*, 28
    vs. oxidation reactions, 30–31, 31t
  hydrolysis in, 26, *26*
  hydroxylation in, *23*, 23–24, 24t
  oxidation reactions in, *23*, 23–24, 24t, *25*
    vs. glucuronide conjugation reactions, 30–31, 31t
  Phase I reactions in, *23*, 23–24, 24t, *25*, 26, *26*, *27*
    vs. Phase II reactions, 30–31, 31t
  Phase II reactions in, 26, *27*, 28, *29*
    vs. Phase I reactions, 30–32, 31t
  reduction reactions in, 24, *26*
  stimulation of, *115*, 115–116, *116*, *117*, 118t

Biotransformation (*Continued*)
  sequential, *27*, *29*, 30, *30*
Body compartments, 7–12, *9*, 10t, *11*
  central, 12
  density of drug molecules in, following intravenous injection, 34, *35*, *36*, 36–37
  intravenous injection of drugs and, volumes of distribution and, 37–38
  one-compartment model, 8–9, *9*
  peripheral, 12
  two-compartment model, *11*, 11–12
    and rapid intravenous injection of drugs, 34, *35*, *36*, 36–37

Clearance, of drugs, and drug interactions, *115*, 115–118, *116*, *117*, 118t
Creatinine clearance, in intravenous injection of drugs, 39–40

Dealkylation, in hepatic biotransformation, 24, 24t, *25*
Drug(s), absorption of, half-life values and, 20
  nonlinear, 92–94, *93*
  accumulation of. See *Drug accumulation.*
  action of, and minimum effective concentration of plasma, *35*, 38–39

Drug(s) (*Continued*)
  active metabolites of, 75–79, 76t, 77, 78
    serum concentrations of, interpretation
      of, 78–79
  and receptor site sensitivity, variations in,
    plasma and serum levels and, 98
  binding of, to proteins. See *Drug-protein
    interaction.*
  clearance of, and drug interactions, 115,
    115–118, 116, 117, 118t
  concentration of, determination of, collec-
    tion of blood samples for, 101–103,
    102
    exponential behavior and, 14–19, 15,
      16, 18
    first-order processes and, 13–19, 15,
      16, 18
    half-life intervals and, 16, 16–17, 18
    half-life values and, interpretation of,
      19–20, 19t
    plasma and serum levels in, 95–103,
      97t, 99, 101t, 102
      clinical usefulness of, 96, 97t
        factors preventing, 97–103, 99,
          101t, 102
      monitoring of, 100–101, 101t
      receptor site disproportionality in, 97
    semilogarithmic plots of, 18, 18–19
  distribution of, and drug interactions, 113,
    114
    body compartments and. See *Body
      compartments.*
    factors influencing, 8
    time and, 34, 35, 36, 36–37
    variations in, plasma and serum levels
      and, 98
    volume of compartments and, 8–11, 9,
      10t
    volumes of, 7–12, 9, 9–10, 10t, 11
  elimination of, 21–32, 23, 24t, 25, 26, 27,
    28t, 29, 30, 31t, 32t. See also *Bio-
    transformation.*
    kidney and, 32, 32t
    liver and, 22–24, 23, 24t, 25, 26, 26,
      27, 28, 28t, 29, 30, 30–31, 31t. See
      also *Biotransformation.*
    routes of, 22
    saturable metabolism and, 90–91
  interaction of. See *Drug interactions.*
  intramuscular, absorption of, completeness
    of, 57
  intramuscular injection of. See *Intramuscu-
    lar injection of drugs.*
  intravenous, action of, and half-life elimi-
    nation, 38–39
    behavior of, time and, 34, 35, 36, 36–
      37
    clearance of, 39–40
      biologic vs. mathematical relationships
        of, 40

Drug(s) (*Continued*)
    intravenous, half-life of elimination and,
      38–39
    intravenous infusion of, 40–42, 41
    intravenous injection of. See *Intravenous
      injection of drugs.*
  loading doses of, drug accumulation and,
    73–74, 74
  metabolism of, impairment of, 116–117,
    118t
  oral, absorption half-life of, 44–47, 46
    absorption of, completeness of, 49–51,
      50
      first-order processes and, 45–47, 46
      rate of, 44–48, 45, 46, 49
        clinical implications of, 48–49, 49
        factors influencing, 47–48
    administration of, 43–52, 45, 46, 49, 50
    bioavailability of, 43–44, 51–52
    rate of absorption of, lag time in, 44, 48
  pharmacokinetics of. See *Pharmacokinet-
    ics.*
  slow-release, 93–94
  therapeutic margin of, 2, 3, 3t
Drug accumulation, accumulation ratio in,
    64–66, 65, 66, 66t
  extent of, 61–68, 62, 64t, 65, 66, 66t, 67
  importance of half-life values in, 71–72,
    71t, 72, 73
  interdose fluctuation in, 67, 67–68
    extent of, 62, 63
  loading doses and, 73–74, 74
  mean steady-state plasma concentration
    and, 62, 62–68, 64t, 65, 66, 66t, 67
  factors influencing, 63–64, 64t
  rate of, 69–74, 70, 71t, 72, 73, 74
Drug dosage, chronic. See *Drug accumula-
    tion.*
Drug interactions, drug clearance and, 115,
    115–118, 116, 117, 118t
  hepatic biotransformation and, 115, 115–
    116, 116, 117, 118t
  pharmacokinetic, 105–109
    and impairment of drug metabolism,
      116–117, 118t
    drug absorption and, 111–113
      completeness of, 112–113
      rate of, 111–112
    drug distribution and, 113, 114
    historical context of, 106
    importance of, 118
    literature on, interpretation of, 108
    mechanisms of, 111–118, 114, 115,
      116, 117, 118t
    renal function and, 117–118
    sources of information on, 106–108
Drug-protein interaction, 81–87, 84t, 86
  factors influencing, 83–84
  free concentration in, vs. free fraction, 82–
    83

Drug-protein interaction (*Continued*)
free fraction in, vs. free concentration, 82–
83
implications of, 84–85
nature of, 81–83
pharmacokinetic data on, interpretation of,
85, *86*
serum concentrations in, 87
variations in, plasma and serum levels
and, 98–100, *99*

Exponential behavior, and drug concentration, 14–19, *15, 16, 18*

First-order process(es), and absorption of
oral drugs, 45–47, *46*
and drug concentration, 13–19, *15, 16,
18*
half-life intervals and, *16,* 16–17, *18*
in nonlinear pharmacokinetics, 89–90
Free concentration (Cf), vs. free fraction, in
drug-protein interaction, 82–83
Free fraction (FF), vs. free concentration, in
drug-protein interaction, 82–83

Glucuronide conjugation reactions, in hepatic
biotransformation, 30–31, 31t
vs. oxidation reactions, *23,* 23–24, 24t, *25*

Half-life values, and absorption of drugs, 20
oral, 44–47, *46*
in drug accumulation, 71–72, 71t, *72, 73*
interpretation of, in drug concentration,
19–20, 19t
Hydrolysis, in hepatic biotransformation, 26,
26
Hydroxylation, in hepatic biotransformation,
23, 23–24, 24t

Intramuscular injection of drugs, 53–60, *55,
56*
adverse effects of, 57
complications of, local, 58–59
systemic, 59
rate of absorption in, physiologic factors
influencing, 56–57
rate of absorption of, physicochemical factors influencing, 54, *55,* 56, *56*
slow, 59

Intravenous injection of drugs, 33–42, *35,
36, 41*
behavior of drugs in, time and, 34, *35, 36,*
36–37
body compartments and, volumes of distribution and, 37–38
creatinine clearance and, 39–40
density of drug molecules after, 34, *35,
36,* 36–37
half-life of elimination and, 38–39
rapid, two-compartment model and, 34,
35, 36, 36–37

Kidney, and elimination of drugs, 32, 32t

Liver, and elimination of drugs, 22–24, *23,*
24t, *25, 26, 26, 27,* 28, 28t, *29, 30,*
30–31, 31t. See also *Biotransformation.*

Metabolism, saturable, and drug elimination,
90–91
in nonlinear pharmacokinetics, 90–91,
91t, *92*
Metabolites, active, drugs with, clinical use
of, 77, 77–79, *78*
pharmacokinetic implications of, 75–79,
76t, 77, *78*
serum concentrations of, interpretation
of, 78–79
therapeutic implications of, 75–79, 76t,
77, *78*
Minimum effective concentration (M.E.C.),
35, 38–39, 48, *49*

Oxidation reactions, in hepatic biotransformation, *23,* 23–24, 24t, *25*
vs. glucuronide conjugation reactions, 30–
31, 31t

Pharmacokinetics, definition of, 4
factors influencing, 4, 5t, 30–31, 31t
limitations of, 5
nonlinear, 89–94, 91t, *92, 93*
first-order processes in, 89–90
saturable metabolism in, 90–91, 91t, *92*
sources of data on, 119–121, 120t
value of, 4

Polypharmacy. See *Drug interactions.*
Prodrugs, *76,* 79
Proteins, binding of drugs to. See *Drug pro-
    tein interaction.*

Reduction reactions, in hepatic biotransfor-
    mation, 24, *26*
Renal function, and pharmacokinetic drug
    interactions, 117–118

Saturable metabolism, and drug elimination,
    90–91
  in nonlinear pharmacokinetics, 90–91, 91t,
    92

Therapeutic margin, and action of drugs, *2,
    3,* 3t

Volumes of distribution, of drugs, 7–12, *9,
    11,* 10t